AN ESSENTIAL
INTRODUCTION TO **CARDIAC**
ELECTROPHYSIOLOGY

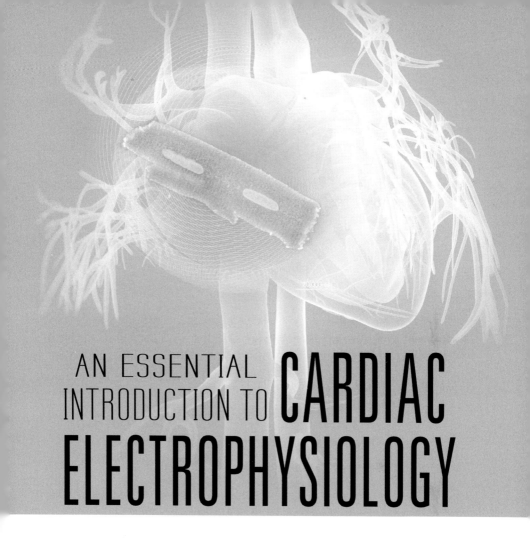

AN ESSENTIAL INTRODUCTION TO CARDIAC
ELECTROPHYSIOLOGY

Ken MacLeod

Imperial College, London, UK

Imperial College Press

ICP

Published by

Imperial College Press
57 Shelton Street
Covent Garden
London WC2H 9HE

Distributed by

World Scientific Publishing Co. Pte. Ltd.
5 Toh Tuck Link, Singapore 596224
USA office: 27 Warren Street, Suite 401-402, Hackensack, NJ 07601
UK office: 57 Shelton Street, Covent Garden, London WC2H 9HE

British Library Cataloguing-in-Publication Data
A catalogue record for this book is available from the British Library.

ISBN 978-1-908977-34-2
ISBN 978-1-908977-35-9 (pbk)

Printed in Singapore by Fulsland Offset Printing (S) Pte Ltd

To my father, Alasdair.

Contents

Preface

The aim of this book is to provide an accessible introduction to cellular cardiac electrophysiology for medical and science students, researchers and aspiring cardiologists. It is largely based on lectures presented to medical and science students undertaking their BSc honours year of study at Imperial College and so the material has been designed chiefly with that level of undergraduate in mind. However, some portions of it will offer sufficient scope for it to be a worthwhile read for postgraduates and it may serve as a useful introductory text for those with doctorates but in allied fields of expertise. The book attempts to overcome the notoriety of the subject being difficult to approach and understand given the complexity of intricate, electrical cellular processes within the human heart.

The book is the result of two students (Ibrahim Ali and Ali Rauf) cajoling me to write something more expansive than the handouts based on my lectures. The subject area has been largely devoid of a successor to Denis Noble's *Initiation of the Heartbeat* published in 1979 and Edward Carmeliet and Johan Vereecke's *Cardiac Cellular Electrophysiology* last published in 2001. While there are a number of multi-author texts, notably Doug Zipes and Jose Jalife's comprehensive and authoritative *Cardiac Electrophysiology: From Cell to Bedside*, all of which cover the ground in excellent detail, they are written for the postgraduate or postdoctoral worker. Ibrahim and Ali recognized the information gap and suggested I start writing. They were to be co-authors, but their medical careers meant that they did not have the time needed to devote to the project.

One of my main objectives when writing the text was to try to describe complex material in a simple way. To do this I had to make a series of judgements about what constituted key material and arbitrate where there is dispute and controversy. In doing so I am well aware that I have omitted descriptions of some important topics and experiments and

xiv   *An Essential Introduction to Cardiac Electrophysiology*

have been a bit offhand (some might say cavalier) with my explanations of those that remain. It is not my intention to be dismissive of a large number of very valuable findings. It is simply because space and time constraints often make it difficult, and sometimes impossible, to report "the complete picture" in this format. I have tried whenever possible to give a balanced and current view, but if that has resulted in some errors of interpretation or omission then the fault lies with me.

Readers will note that throughout the book I have been parsimonious with the use of references. This is because it is not my intention to catalogue an array of experimental detail, but rather to provide a framework within which readers can discover their own interests and upon which they can build their own bibliography. At the end of each chapter I have detailed a number of reviews and texts that provide initial "way points" and in some cases I have supplemented these with references to original papers that are either in the "classic" category or provide salient information.

There are two superb texts that I would recommend reading in conjunction with this one because they cover areas I have deliberately avoided. I have not described in detail how an ECG arises, or discussed the diagnostic significance of its various waveforms, nor have I covered excitation–contraction coupling in cardiac muscle, even though these could be deemed to fall within the subject area of this book. Arnold Katz's *Physiology of the Heart* is a landmark monograph which meticulously covers whole heart physiology and biochemistry. Don Bers' *Excitation–Contraction Coupling and Cardiac Contractile Force* is a readable and very comprehensive description of cardiac contraction which has set a high standard for balancing thorough detail with readability. I would hope this more meagre offering supplements these in some small way. I am optimistic that readers will feel more confident and at ease with electrical concepts and the important physiological mechanisms that govern the initiation and regulation of the heartbeat.

I have been helped along the way by a variety of friends and colleagues. My grateful thanks to Markus Sikkel who has read and commented on the whole book so now needs to lie down in a dark room for while. To the others I offer a variety of quotes.

To the many students I have taught over the years:

> I learned very early the difference between knowing the name of something and knowing something. Richard Feynman

To my many friends:

> Outside of a dog, a book is man's best friend. Inside of a dog it's too dark to read. Groucho Marx

To Jackie Downs at Imperial College Press:

> I love deadlines. I love the whooshing noise they make as they go by. Douglas Adams

To my wife and companion in life, Wendy:

> Those who have never known the deep intimacy and the intense companionship of happy mutual love have missed the best thing that life has to give. Bertrand Russell

I end with another quote from Richard Feynman. He was a theoretical physicist who received the Nobel Prize in Physics in 1965 for his work in quantum electrodynamics, a subject area that describes how light and matter interact. Feynman was not only a profound thinker, but also a raconteur admired for his ability to explain difficult concepts with humour and wonderful analogies. Using these talents he popularized what is still a conceptually difficult area of physics.

> We are at the very beginning of time for the human race. It is not unreasonable that we grapple with problems. But there are tens of thousands of years in the future. Our responsibility is to do what we can, learn what we can, improve the solutions, and pass them on.

I suppose this book is my way of doing just that.

Ken MacLeod
London, 2013

Chapter 1

Introduction

1.1 Early references to the heart and its function

Reference to the heart being associated with the transport of blood was noted in an Egyptian papyrus dating from around 1550 BC (Papyrus Ebers). The Egyptians observed that the heart was connected to many vessels that seemingly carried many different kinds of body fluid. About 1000 years later, the heart, its valves and the blood vessels attached to it were more fully described by Hippocrates and his students but their precise functions remained uncertain. Blood vessels were thought to carry air around the body, and when they were cut and bled it was supposed that the air was being replaced by blood which had leaked from the organs. Aristotle reasoned that the heart formed part of the soul because it is centrally located in the body, is essential for life, all animals have one and it appears to be affected by emotion.

> For it is in the front and centre of the body that the heart is situated, in which we say is the principle of life and the source of all motion and sensation.

By the second century AD it was known that there were two types of blood vessels, arteries and veins, and that the arterial blood contained dissolved gases. An eminent Greek physician of the time, called Aelius Galenus or Galen, thought that the arterial blood was created in the heart and that the arteries pushed blood through them due to their own pulsatile properties and not by the action of the heart. Blood was consumed by the organs of the body and did not return to the heart. He wrote,

1

...it is quite evident that the heart is a part of the vessels and their origin; and for this it is well suited by its structure. For its central part consists of a dense and hollow substance, and is moreover full of blood, as though the vessels took thence their origin. It is hollow to serve for the reception of the blood, while its wall is dense...For the blood is conveyed into the vessels from the heart, but none passes into the heart from without. For in itself it constitutes the origin and fountain, or primary receptacle, of the blood. ...For the motions of the body commence from the heart, and are brought about by traction and relaxation. The heart therefore, ...[is]...a living creature inside its possessor.

With innate accuracy, Leonardo da Vinci's illustrations of the heart in the 15th century show an understanding that it has four chambers and that the valves permit the flow of blood only in one direction. However, da Vinci was more concerned with anatomical exactness rather than understanding precise function, and clung to the earlier ideas that the blood was transported to the other organs where it would be used up. It was not until William Harvey, an English physician, published his treatise in 1628 entitled *On the Motion of the Heart and Blood in Animals* that the function of the heart and its relationship with the circulation was correctly described. Harvey wrote,

From these and other observations of a similar nature, I am persuaded it will be found that the motion of the heart is as follows:

First of all, the auricle contracts, and in the course of its contraction forces the blood (which it contains in ample quantity as the head of the veins, the store-house and cistern of the blood) into the ventricle, which, being filled, the heart raises itself straightway, makes all its fibres tense, contracts the ventricles, and performs a beat, by which beat it immediately sends the blood supplied to it by the auricle into the arteries. The right ventricle sends its charge into the lungs by the vessel which is called vena arteriosa, but which in structure and function, and all other respects, is an artery. The left ventricle sends its charge into the aorta, and through this by the arteries to the body at large.

The motion of the heart, then, is entirely of this description, and the one action of the heart is the transmission of the blood and its distribution, by means of the arteries, to the very extremities of the body; so that the pulse which we feel in the arteries is nothing more than the impulse of the blood derived from the heart.

I began to think whether there might not be a motion, as it were, in a circle. Now, this I afterwards found to be true; and I finally saw that the blood, forced by the action of the left ventricle into the arteries, was distributed to the body at large, and its several parts, in the same manner as it is sent through the lungs, impelled by the right ventricle into the pulmonary artery, and that it then passed through the veins and along the vena cava, and so round to the left ventricle in the manner already indicated. This motion we may be allowed to call circular...

Harvey had correctly identified the function the heart and that of the circulation, but the notion that the contraction of the heart was a result of its intrinsic electrical properties was not realized until several hundred years later.

1.2 Early references to electrical properties

That muscles had electrical properties associated with their contraction was arguably first demonstrated by Luigi Galvani around 1791, but it was not until the invention and development of the galvanometer (an instrument that could detect electric current) that heart muscle contraction was observed by Julius Bernstein and Theodor Wilhelm Engelmann around 1875 to be accompanied by an electrical impulse, which occurred before the contractile event and was propagated from the site of stimulation across the ventricles. Arguments developed about whether the heartbeat was initiated within the tissue itself or was the consequence of its innervation. Around the same time, Walter Gaskell was also investigating the sequence of contraction of the isolated, slowly beating tortoise heart preparation. Gaskell found that the contractions started in the sinus venosus and, in an almost peristaltic motion, transferred to the equivalent of the atrium and then to the ventricle. The rhythmical beating occurred independently of innervation and always appeared to start in the sinus venosus, an area of the heart that we would regard today as containing the pacemaker. These discoveries were supported by Arthur Keith and Martin Flack who, in 1907, pinpointed the area of human heart responsible for the initiation of the impulse – the sino-atrial node.

The velocity and direction of propagation were investigated more fully by John Burdon Sanderson and Frederick Page in 1880, and then in 1887 Augustus Waller made the first recordings of the electrical activity of the heart using electrodes placed externally, first on the chest, then on the arms. Waller was sceptical that his recordings of these electrical events would be useful, but was encouraged and helped by the interest of the physiologists Willem Einthoven and Thomas Lewis.

Einthoven made several modifications to the galvanometer, and around 1895 started to use three combinations of recording electrode (on the right and left hand, on the right hand and left foot and on the left hand and left foot), which became the standard "Einthoven leads". In 1906 he wrote a detailed paper in which he described consistent features of electrocardiographical recordings from patients with different heart conditions. Thomas Lewis was interested in studying cardiac arrhythmias but he realized that to do it effectively he needed to be able to see and compare recordings of the electrical activity of the hearts of his patients. From about 1908 he corresponded with Einthoven regularly, and he is credited with being responsible for introducing electrocardiograph (ECG) machines into hospital practice and illustrating that these could help diagnose a variety of conditions of the heart.

1.3 The electrocardiograph

During each beat of the heart a wave of depolarization spreads through its cells in a coordinated and synchronized way. Einthoven used the fact that the body is a good conductor of electricity and found that these changes in electrical activity could be detected as small increases and decreases in voltage between two electrodes placed on the limbs of a patient. In electrocardiography usually an electrode is connected to each wrist and ankle, with the one on the right foot serving as a zero volt reference point and the remaining three used as the recording electrodes. The electrode positions correspond to three points of an equilateral triangle (called Einthoven's triangle) with the heart lying at its centre surrounded by homogeneously conducting body tissues (Fig. 1.1). The three electrodes can be connected together in different combinations – called leads – to record the ECG. Each lead reports the electrical activity of the heart from a different angle in one plane (called the frontal plane). Einthoven assigned the letters P, Q, R, S and T to the various voltage deflections.

Each beat of the heart (the cardiac cycle) is initiated by depolarization at the sino-atrial node that spreads across the atria. The first electrical signal recorded by the ECG comes from the atria and is called the P wave. The wave of depolarization activates contraction of the atria that tops up the ventricles with blood. When compared with ventricular tissue the muscle mass of the atria is relatively small so, correspondingly, the amplitude of the P wave is small (Fig. 1.1). After the P wave, the ECG recording returns to the baseline for a short interval caused by a slowing of the conduction of the impulse between the atria and ventricles. This slowing of conduction means that the atria can contract fully and fill the ventricles with blood before the ventricles themselves are stimulated. The next change in the ECG trace is called the QRS complex and is caused by depolarization of the septum and ventricles (Fig. 1.1). The depolarization activates ventricular contraction which is initially isometric (non-shortening) producing an increase in pressure in both chambers (isovolumetric contraction). This is followed by a phase of isotonic (shortening) contraction which ejects the blood once pressure in the left and right ventricles exceeds that in the aorta and pulmonary artery respectively. Blood is pumped from the chambers. Since the muscle mass of the ventricles is larger than that of the atria, the QRS complex is much larger than the P wave. By convention, the first upward deflection is always called the R wave, regardless of whether or not it has been preceded by a downward-going Q wave. Any deflection going below the baseline immediately after the R wave is called the S wave.

The volume of blood ejected decreases and the ventricular muscle relaxes (isovolumetric relaxation). This phase corresponds with a further deflection on the ECG trace called the T wave. This is caused by

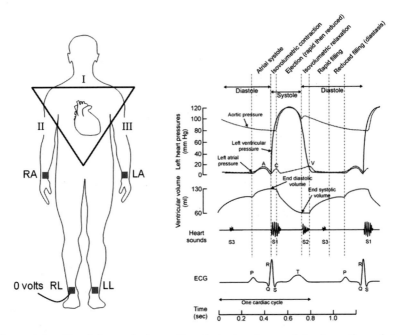

Figure 1.1.   The left panel shows the electrode placement to form the points of Einthoven's triangle and the recording leads I, II and III. Lead I records the voltage between the (positive) left arm (LA) electrode and right arm (RA) electrode. Lead II records the voltage between the (positive) left leg (LL) electrode and the right arm (RA) electrode. Lead III records the voltage between the (positive) left leg (LL) electrode and the left arm (LA) electrode. The right panel illustrates the phases of the cardiac cycle with the corresponding ECG changes in the form of a diagram established by Carl Wiggers.

repolarization of the ventricles. At this time the ventricles start to fill with blood again and the cardiac cycle is repeated (Fig. 1.1).

Although the depolarization that generates the QRS complex spreads across both ventricles, it has a mean direction or vector that is usually towards the left ventricle because of its greater muscle mass. However, the precise direction of this mean frontal plane axis depends on the anatomical orientation of the heart in the chest and the relative masses of the two ventricles. The direction of the mean frontal plane axis can therefore change (e.g. if a portion of the left ventricular muscle dies following myocardial infarction or the chamber walls enlarge) and so its direction can be an important sign of cardiac pathology.

In addition, because of their placement, the leads will show a different form of the ECG, even though their signals all come from the same source. Some leads will have a predominantly positive-going QRS complex whilst others will have predominantly negative QRS complexes. By examining these different waveforms it is possible to diagnose abnormal rhythms and identify areas of the heart where there is damage to the conductive tissue that carries the electrical signals.

1.4 Cellular electrophysiology

Investigations of cardiac excitation processes remained comparatively quiescent until 1949, when Silvio Weidmann started to make intracellular recordings of the cardiac action potential using a microelectrode made from a glass capillary that had a tip small enough to penetrate the muscle cells without injury. Improvements in the technique of making and filling such microelectrodes by G.N. Ling, who was a graduate student of Professor R.W. Gerard in Chicago, were fundamental to its introduction and then widespread use as a major electrophysiological research tool.

Weidmann recalled that he

> became a heart physiologist by 2-fold chance: from 5 to 6 p.m. Dr. Feldberg had demonstrated a Starling preparation to the medical students and allowed me [access to the] heart; and my wife agreed that I need not be home for supper at 6:30.

Both he and his wife must be credited with laying the foundations of cardiac cell electrophysiology.

1.5 Heart anatomy and location

The adult heart is about 12 cm in length and about 8 cm in width. In males it weighs between 280 and 340 g and in females between 230 and

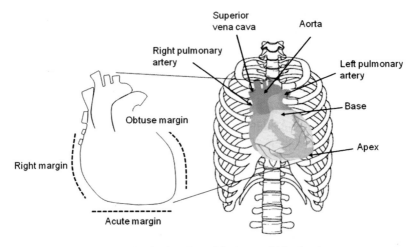

Figure 1.2. The location of the heart within the chest.

280 g. It has four chambers, the right and left atria and the right and left ventricles. The atria are separated from the ventricles at the coronary sulcus, an external groove also termed the atrioventricular groove, on the outer surface of the heart in which run the coronary arteries and veins. The left ventricle is separated from the right ventricle by the interventricular septum.

The base of the heart is formed mainly by the left atrium and a portion of the right atrium and lies separated from the fifth to eighth thoracic vertebrae by the oesophagus and aorta. The apex of the heart points to the left when the heart is viewed as it lies within the body and is situated behind the fifth left intercostal space, 8 to 9 cm from the mid-sternal line (Fig. 1.2).

The right ventricle forms the sternocostal surface while the diaphragmatic surface is formed by both ventricles. The right boundary (or margin) of the heart is formed by the right atrium above and the right ventricle below and is situated behind the third to fifth right costal cartilages about 1 cm from the sternal margin. The lower boundary, called the acute margin, is virtually horizontal and is formed by the ventricles. It extends from the sternal end of the sixth right costal cartilage to the apex. The left boundary (called the obtuse margin) is the shortest of the three margins and formed mainly by the left ventricle. It extends from the second left intercostal space near the sternal margin to the apex. In most cases, about two-thirds of the heart lies to the left of the midline of the sternum with the other third positioned to the right of the midline.

The left ventricle forms the apex of the heart. Its walls are about three times as thick as those of the right ventricle. Attached to the internal walls of the ventricle are densely interlaced muscle strands called trabeculae, some of which are fixed at their ends with the middle part free-running and others are attached along their entire length. A third type of trabeculae, the papillary muscles, are thicker and attached to the ventricular walls at one end but have a free end from which originate thin but tough tendons called chordae tendonae. There are two papillary muscles, and separately their tendons attach to the anterior and posterior cusps of the mitral valve. These prevent the cusps prolapsing into the left atrium during the systolic phases of the cardiac cycle.

The right ventricle extends from the right atrium to near the apex of the heart. The free wall of the right ventricle is thinner than that of the left and the trabeculae are less dense. There are three papillary muscles in the right ventricle and these individually are attached to the anterior, posterior and septal leaflets of the tricuspid valve. They perform a similar function as those on the left side of the heart preventing prolapse of the tricuspid valve leaflets during systole.

The inside lining of the chambers is continuous with the lining of the large blood vessels. This layer, called the endocardium, consists of connective tissue covered by endothelial cells and contains blood vessels and nerves. Fibrous rings surround the entry points of the blood vessels to the heart. These rings provide anchoring for the blood vessels and the mitral, tricuspid and semilunar valves.

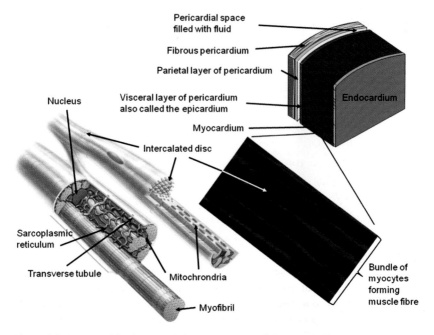

Figure 1.3. Layers of the heart and the components of the ventricular myocyte. Some of the components will be discussed in much more detail in later chapters.

The outermost layer of the heart is called the epicardium and is the serous layer of the pericardium. Between the epi- and endocardium is the myocardium (Fig. 1.3). About 3 billion myocytes or muscle cells make up the human myocardium and, while they constitute the main mass of the heart in terms of cell volume and protein, they are greatly outnumbered by other cell types. In terms of numbers, about 30% of the heart comprises myocytes, 64% fibroblasts and 6% endothelial and smooth muscle cells. The endothelial and smooth muscle cells arise from the blood vessels serving the heart itself. Fibroblasts are a type of cell that produces the extracellular matrix, the structural framework for animal tissues.

The myocytes are joined together to form bundles of muscle fibres which are arranged in a complex way to create the chambers. Atrial fibre bundles are arranged in two layers. The outermost layer is common to both chambers while the deeper, inner layer is distinct for each. The

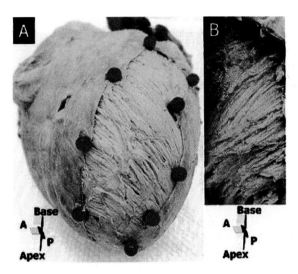

Figure 1.4. An example of the spiral arrangement of muscle fibres in the left ventricle of a pig heart. The directon of fibre alignment changes from a left-handed spiral in the sub-epicardium (Panel A) to a right-handed spiral in the sub-endocardium (Panel B). The orientation of the preparations can be assessed using the small axes below the illustrations (A, anterior; P, posterior). Reproduced with permission from Sengupta *et al.* (2006) *J. Amer. Coll. Cardiol.* **48**, 1988–2001.

deep layers consist of loops of muscle fibres that form the walls and "roof" of each atrial chamber. They are attached at each end to the atrioventricular ring. Ventricular muscle fibres are also arranged in surface and deep layers. These twist, spiralling in clockwise and anti-clockwise directions. However, there is a gradual continuum of fibre orientation across the ventricular wall from the clockwise spiral in the sub-endocardial region to the anti-clockwise helix in the sub-epicardial region (Fig. 1.4).

Modern imaging techniques such as high-resolution echocardiography and magnetic resonance imaging show the regional and global movement of the heart during the cardiac cycle to be very complex. Shortening of the inner sub-endocardial fibres is concomitant with stretching of the outer sub-epicardial fibres. During contraction, the spiralling of the fibre orientation causes rotation of the heart particularly at the apex. During the isovolumic contraction phase the apex undergoes

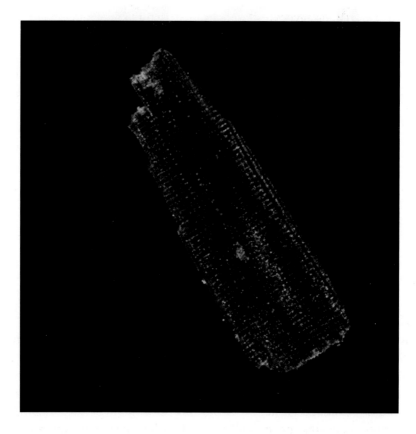

Figure 1.5.   An isolated ventricular myocyte. The cell is 120 μm long and 36 μm wide. Ventricular myocytes usually have two nuclei (here stained with DAPI (4',6-diamidino-2-phenylindole), a fluorescent stain that binds to DNA and produces a blue colour). The cell has a striated appearance because it is also labelled with α-actinin antibodies. α-actinin attaches actin filaments to the Z-line of the sarcomere. I am grateful to Dr. Anita Alvarez Laviada in my laboratory for providing this image.

clockwise rotation corresponding with initial activation of the sub-endocardial fibres, but during the rapid ejection phase the apical rotation reverses and is anti-clockwise, which corresponds with slightly later activation of the sub-epicardial fibres. The sequential activation of the different chambers and muscle fibres requires coordinated electrical stimulation via discrete conduction pathways which will be described in Chapter 8.

The ventricular myocyte is roughly rectangular in shape, about 150 μm long and 25 μm wide (Figs. 1.4 and 1.5). About 46% of the volume of the ventricular myocyte is composed of myofibrils – the contractile elements of the cell. As an indication of the high energy demands of these cells, the mitochondria occupy about 38% of the volume of the cell and are located next to the myofibrils. Each myofibril stretches the length of the cell and is anchored at each end at fasciae adherens junctions, which bind cells together and transmit the contractile force.

It is how these cells are electrically excited and the molecular mechanisms that underlie the excitation process that is the main focus of this book.

1.6 How this book is organized

The book chapters ought to be read in numerical order. Chapters 2 to 5 provide a large amount of necessary background material for the two main chapters (Chapters 6 and 7) that describe the trans-membrane electrical events that shape the ventricular action potential. Chapter 2 illustrates how the resting membrane potential is formed. Understanding this process is fundamental to appreciating how ionic movements across membranes produce voltage changes. In Chapter 3 some of the elementary concepts of electricity are explained with reference to excitable cells. These explanations are followed by a short description of pioneering experiments carried out in the 1940s and 1950s that measured current flow across nerve cell membranes. Although not on cardiac tissue, it is important to appreciate the experimental procedures used and the concepts proposed at that time because they lay the foundations for the experimental and analytical approaches we use today when trying to understand the trans-membrane events that occur during the cardiac action potential. Chapter 4 explains recent experimental techniques and proposals about how ion channels function, with emphasis on the relationship between protein structure and function. Chapter 5 similarly examines the important ion exchangers and ion pumps involved in cardiac excitation. The currents flowing during the ventricular action potential are described in detail in Chapters 6 and 7. Chapter 6 focuses on the important features of the early parts of the ventricular action potential and explains, in terms of the currents that flow during it, the underlying electrical events. Chapter 7 describes the currents that flow during the later parts of the ventricular action potential. To illustrate the differences and similarities between the excitatory process in cells from opposite ends of the excitation process, Chapter 8 describes the ionic currents flowing in sino-atrial cells, the cardiac pacemaker. Lastly, Chapter 9 illustrates the excitatory processes that may change to give rise to arrhythmias and briefly reviews the pharmaceutical interventions that can be used to overcome aberrant excitatory processes. Every chapter begins with a check list of key points that will be covered and ends with a summary of the material. Questions are then provided to test understanding. Scattered throughout the book are blue boxes that can be skipped if the reader wishes. They contain background or extra information designed to add a further aspect to the main details.

Some heart facts

In a year, the heart pumps 2.5 million litres of blood. Equivalent to the volume of an Olympic-sized swimming pool.

Assuming a person is not performing any great amount of physical activity, their heart beats about 36.5 million times per year.

During each beat all the heart tissue becomes electrically activated within 230 ms.

The heart can respond to the needs of the body by being able to increase its output at least four times from 5 l.min^{-1} to 22 l.min^{-1}.

The heart performs a large amount of work so has a high demand for oxygen. Again, assuming a person is not performing any great amount of physical activity, their heart alone uses 16,000 litres of oxygen per year, roughly equivalent to the volume of 225 car tanks of petrol (assuming the volume of an average tank is 60 litres).

1.7 Bibliography

Burdon-Sanderson, J. and Page, F.J.M. (1880). On the time-relations of the excitatory process in the ventricle of the heart of the frog. *J. Physiol.* **2**, 384–435.

Einthoven W. (1906). Le telecardiogramme. *Arch. Int. Physiol.* **4**:132–164 (translated into English by Blackburn, H.W. (1957). *Amer. Heart J.* **53**, 602–615).

Electronic Scholarly Publishing (2000). *On the Natural Faculties.* Galen (170). Translated by Brock, A.J. [Online] Available at: www.esp.org/books/galen/natural-faculties/html/title.html.

Engelmann, T. (1878). Ueber das electrische verhalten des thätigen herzens. *Pflügers Archiv.* **17**, 68–99.

Gaskell, W.H. (1883). On the innervation of the heart, with special reference to the heart of the tortoise. *J. Physiol.* **4**, 43–127.

Internet Classics Archive (1994). *On the Parts of Animals.* Aristotle (350 BC). Translated by Ogle, W. [Online]
Available at: http://classics.mit.edu/Aristotle/parts_animals.html.

Keele, K.D. (1951). Leonardo da Vinci, and the movement of the heart. *Proc. R. Soc. Med.* **44**, 209–213.

Keith, A. and Flack, M. (1907). The form and nature of the muscular connections between the primary divisions of the vertebrate heart. *J. Anat. Physiol.* **41**, 172–189.

Lewis, T. (1907). The interpretation of the primary and first secondary wave in sphygmograph tracings. *J. Anat. Physiol.* **41**, 137–140.

Open Library (2008). *Exercitatio Anatomica de Motu Cordis et Sanguinis in Animalibus.* Harvey, W. (1628). Translated by Leake, C.D. (1928). [Online] Available at:

http://openlibrary.org/books/OL13506205M/Exercitatio_anatomica_de_ motu_cordis_et_sanguinis_in_animalibus.

The Papyrus Ebers. Translated by Bryan, C.P. (1930) [Online] Available at:
http://oilib.uchicago.edu/books/bryan_the_papyrus_ebers_1930.pdf.

Waller, A. (1887). A demonstration in man of electromotive changes accompanying the heart's beat. *J. Physiol.* **8**, 229–234.

Weidmann, S. (1961). Membrane excitation in cardiac muscle. *Circulation* **24**, 499–505.

Chapter 2

The Resting Membrane Potential

The resting membrane potential is the voltage difference between the inside and outside of the cell. It arises from the movement of ions across the plasma membrane, which results from the operation of ion channels, pumps and other forms of ion transporter. The term "resting membrane potential" of an excitable cell refers to the period between action potentials when the cell is electrically quiescent.

2.1 Chapter objectives

After reading this chapter you should:
- Understand how the membrane potential is generated
- Know the meaning of the term "equilibrium potential"
- Be able to calculate equilibrium potentials in simple systems using the Nernst equation
- Realize that the E_m is usually determined by potassium ion flux
- Understand the underlying principles quantitatively described by the Goldman–Hodgkin–Katz equation
- Be able to assess the contribution of pumped ionic fluxes to the membrane potential

2.2 How is the resting membrane potential generated?

The plasma membrane plays an important role in establishing the resting membrane potential since it sets up a selective barrier to the movement of charged species. The ease with which charged species cross the barrier depends on its permeability to them and this differs between cell types and during the physiological functions of the cell. Trans-membrane movement of charge is also dependent on the ionic composition of the cell cytoplasm differing from that of the extracellular fluid. The differences in concentration of various molecular species across the membrane prime their movement (or flux), and the principle whereby such species flow from regions of high to low concentration is called *diffusion*. The generation (and magnitude) of the membrane potential of a cardiac muscle cell is due to the unequal separation of charged species across the plasma membrane.

To help understand how the membrane potential is generated consider the simple experimental set-up outlined below in Fig. 2.1. There are two chambers separated by an impermeable membrane (Fig. 2.1 Panel A). Two different concentrations of potassium chloride (KCl) are added to each compartment – say 100 mM in the left chamber and 10 mM in the right. A voltmeter allows us to measure any potential difference that forms across the membrane. In this condition, there is obviously a concentration gradient across the membrane (from chamber 1 to 2) but since it is impermeable to any ions, no potential difference between the chambers is generated.

We now change the characteristics of the membrane by incorporating some K^+ channels within it so that it is now permeable *only* to K^+ ions, as shown in Fig. 2.1 Panel B. The change in membrane permeability allows the process of diffusion to occur and there is net movement of ions from a region of higher concentration to one of lower concentration, as indicated by the red arrow designating the *concentration gradient*. K^+ ions diffuse carrying positive charge with them. Positive charge accumulates in chamber 2 as it gains cations whilst chamber 1 loses cations. As electrical charge builds up in chamber 2, an *electrical gradient* forms (designated by the blue arrow), which tends to oppose the movement of ions driven by the concentration difference (Fig. 2.1 Panel C). Although the concentration difference still drives the movement of K^+ ions from chamber 1 to chamber 2, at the same time their passage is

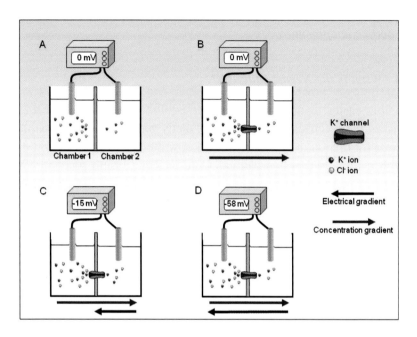

Figure 2.1. Panel A: The set-up to record potential difference between two solutions separated by an impermeable membrane. Panel B: The membrane is now permeable to K^+ ions and they diffuse according to the concentration gradient (red arrow). Panel C: K^+ ions carry positive charge which accumulates in chamber 2. As electrical charge builds up in chamber 2, an electrical gradient forms (blue arrow), which tends to oppose the movement of ions driven by the concentration gradient. Panel D: Equilibrium is reached when the electrical gradient between the two chambers exactly balances the concentration gradient. If there is a ten-fold difference in K^+ ion concentration between the two chambers the equilibrium will be reached when chamber 2 is 58 mV more positive than chamber 1 (at room temperature).

being repelled by the increasing positive charge in chamber 2. The electrical difference between the two chambers builds up until it exactly balances the concentration difference and an *equilibrium* is reached (Fig. 2.1 Panel D). The probability that a K^+ ion will move from chamber 1 to chamber 2 is the same as the probability it will move in the reverse direction and so there is no further net movement of K^+. In other words, K^+ ions will still move but the same number will leave chamber 1 as arrive from chamber 2. At this point the charge (or electrical) difference exactly balances the concentration (or chemical) difference between the two chambers and the voltage measured across the membrane is called the *equilibrium potential*.

2.2.1 *What is the Nernst equation?*

It is now easier to understand that the equilibrium potential of an ion describes the electrical potential that exactly balances the concentration gradient for the ion in question. If we know the concentrations of the ion in both chambers then we can calculate its equilibrium potential (E_{ion}) using the *Nernst equation*:

$$E_{ion} = \frac{RT}{zF} \ln \frac{[ion]_1}{[ion]_2} \qquad (2.1)$$

with:

E	equilibrium potential of ionic species (volts (V))
R	gas constant ($8.314 \ J.K^{-1}mol^{-1}$)
T	absolute temperature (Kelvin (K))
z	valence of ion
F	Faraday constant ($96\ 485 \ C.mol^{-1}$)
$\ln$	logarithm to base e
$[ion]_1$	concentration of ion in chamber 1
$[ion]_2$	concentration of ion in chamber 2

A slightly easier form of the equation can be obtained by partially solving it using the constants, converting the natural logarithm to the common logarithm ($\log_{10}$) and assuming the system is at 37 °C. The Nernst equation then becomes:

$$E_{ion} = \frac{61}{z} \log \frac{[ion]_1}{[ion]_2} \qquad (2.2)$$

Equations 2.1 and 2.2 relate the size of the equilibrium potential of an ion to the size of its concentration gradient. For instance, the larger the concentration gradient, the larger the equilibrium potential will be, because a larger electrically driven movement of ions will be required to balance the movement of ions due to the concentration difference. Note that a ten-fold difference in concentration of the ion across a membrane selectively permeable to that ion will produce $61/z$ mV of potential difference.

In a more physiological situation we tend to express E in millivolts and define chamber 1 as the outside of the cell and chamber 2 as the inside. If there is a ten-fold difference of K^+ across the membrane the potential will be −61 mV.

Derivation of the Nernst equation

A straightforward way of thinking about how the Nernst equation is derived is to try to appreciate what driving forces underlie the existence of the equilibrium potential and if these are favourable or not. A quantity known as the Gibbs free energy (G) of the system reflects the balance between such forces. The free energy change associated with moving a mole of ion X at a higher concentration in one chamber X_1 across a plasma membrane to a lower concentration X_2 in another chamber is:

$$\Delta G_{conc} = RT \ln \frac{[X]_1}{[X]_2}$$

The free energy change associated with moving a mole of a charged particle with valence z in an electrical field E is:

$$\Delta G_{elect} = zFE$$

When the ionic species is at equilibrium across the membrane the free energies balance:

$$\Delta G_{conc} = \Delta G_{elect}$$

So:

$$RT \ln \frac{[X]_1}{[X]_2} = zFE$$

$$\Leftrightarrow E = \frac{RT}{zF} \ln \frac{[X]_1}{[X]_2}$$

2.2.2 *How does changing the potential difference affect ion flow?*

It is possible for the electrical potential to overcome an ionic concentration difference. In fact, many electrophysiological studies take advantage of our ability to alter ion flux by changing either the electrical potential across the membrane or the concentration of important ions on either side of the membrane. To understand how changing the potential difference across the cell membrane can alter ion movement across it, we can take the example of the two chambers in Fig. 2.2 Panel A and connect a battery across the membrane to control the electrical potential without interfering with the initial distribution of ions in the two chambers. We suppose the small battery generates 100 mV. Whilst the battery is not switched on, there will be a flux of K^+ from chamber 1 to chamber 2 causing a membrane potential to develop with chamber 1 being negative with respect to chamber 2. If the battery is now switched into the circuit, making chamber 1 initially much more negative (-161 mV) than chamber 2 (Fig. 2.2 Panel B), the K^+ flux will be reversed because the positive K^+ ions will be attracted to the negative potential of chamber 1. The electrical difference is now greater than the concentration difference and K^+ ions will flow against the latter until a new equilibrium is achieved. Correspondingly, if the battery polarity is reversed, the electrical difference $(+39 \text{ mV})$ is now less than the concentration difference and more K^+ ions will move from chamber 1 to chamber 2 than when no battery was in the circuit. A new equilibrium will be established (Fig. 2.2 Panel C). Therefore, both the direction and magnitude of ion flux depend on the membrane potential (see Fig. 2.2 Panel D).

2.3 K^+ ion and the membrane potential

In most excitable cells – and heart cells are no exception – the ion that contributes most significantly to the resting membrane potential is K^+. There is a larger intracellular K^+ concentration (about 120 mM) compared with the normal extracellular K^+ concentration (about 4 mM) and the membrane is highly permeable to this cation compared with

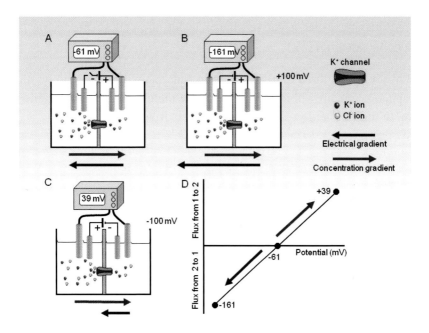

Figure 2.2. Panel A: A similar example to the set-up in Fig. 2.1 except this experiment is done at 37 °C and a battery is introduced across the membrane to control the electrical potential without interfering with the initial distribution of ions in the two chambers. The small battery generates 100 mV. Whilst the battery is not switched on, the flux of K^+ ions from chamber 1 to chamber 2 causes a membrane potential to develop. Panel B: The battery is now switched into the circuit, making chamber 1 initially more negative (−161 mV) than chamber 2. The electrical difference (blue arrow) is now greater than the concentration difference (red arrow) and K^+ ions will flow against the latter until a new equilibrium is achieved. Panel C: The battery polarity is reversed compared with the experimental system in Panel B. The electrical difference (+39 mV) is now less than the concentration difference and more K^+ ions will move from chamber 1 to chamber 2 compared with when no battery was in the circuit. Panel D: The direction and size of the ion movements depend on the membrane potential. In this case E_K occurs at −61 mV. Any positive change in membrane potential (i.e. in the depolarizing direction) will force a movement of K^+ ions from chamber 1 to chamber 2 and a negative change in membrane potential (i.e. in the hyperpolarizing direction) will force a movement of K^+ ions from chamber 2 to chamber 1.

other ions at rest. As a result, K^+ ions will tend to diffuse out of the cell down its concentration gradient. In terms of the total number of ions in a cell, only a small percentage cross the membrane (see Info Box "How many ions move?" on p. 30), but sufficient to create a separation of charge, leaving a net negative charge inside the cell so producing the membrane potential (E_m).

The major intracellular anions, which include many proteins and organic phosphates, remain within the cell since the membrane is impermeable to them. In this case $E_m = -90$ mV calculated as follows:

$$E_K = \frac{61}{1} \log \frac{4}{120} = -90\text{mV} \qquad (2.3)$$

This is also the K^+ equilibrium potential (E_K). E_m usually lies very close to the value of E_K.

2.3.1 *What are the equilibrium potentials for other ions in the heart?*

The same calculations can be made for any other ion (see Table 2.1). For example, if the membrane were uniquely permeable to Na^+ and the concentrations of the ion on either side of it were as detailed in Table 2.1, then the potential across the membrane would be +70 mV. If no other ion is present the equilibrium potential can also be called the *reversal potential* (E_{rev}) since this is the potential at which the overall direction of ion flux reverses.

2.3.2 *How do other ions contribute to the resting potential?*

If we measured the actual membrane potential existing across the plasma membrane of a ventricular muscle cell we would find that it is about −80 mV and less negative than E_K. We know that, given the appropriate intracellular and extracellular concentrations of K^+ and a membrane only permeable to K^+, the membrane potential should equal E_K. This would be the case in an ideal system but the biological reality is that the cell has a small permeability to other ions, notably Na^+, Ca^{2+} and Cl^-. This means that the resting membrane potential is generally more positive than the predicted E_K value. To appreciate the influence of other ion

Ion	[extracellular] (mM)	[intracellular] (mM)	E_{ion} (mV)	Relative permeability at rest (P_X/P_K)
K^+	4	120	-90	1.00
Na^+	140	10	$+70$	0.04
Ca^{2+}	2	100×10^{-4}	$+131$	0.20
Cl^-	100	22	-40	0.11

Table 2.1. Equilibrium potentials (E_{ion}) for important ions in the heart.

permeabilities, consider the following Figures 2.3–2.6 in which the membrane is permeable to K^+ and Na^+ at various times.

In Fig. 2.3 there are ten-fold K^+ and Na^+ concentration differences across the membrane and initially K^+ channels are open but Na^+ channels are shut. The membrane potential can be calculated to be –61 mV. Remember this is also E_K at these ionic concentrations. Now consider Fig. 2.4, which illustrates a similar set-up but this time K^+ channels are shut and Na^+ channels are open. The membrane potential is now +61 mV which is also E_{Na}. If both types of channel are now open the membrane is permeable to both K^+ and Na^+ equally. Figure 2.5 shows that each ion diffuses according to its concentration difference and the membrane potential produced is not at either equilibrium potential but lies half-way between the two equilibrium potentials, at 0 mV. If there is now unequal permeability such that there are three times as many K^+ channels as Na^+ channels (as in Fig. 2.6), then the membrane is much more permeable to K^+ so the membrane potential moves towards E_K. However, there is a finite permeability of the membrane to Na^+ so the membrane potential is also influenced and drawn towards E_{Na}. The final membrane potential settles at a value weighted towards E_K, the weighting being dependent on the relative permeability and concentration of each ion species.

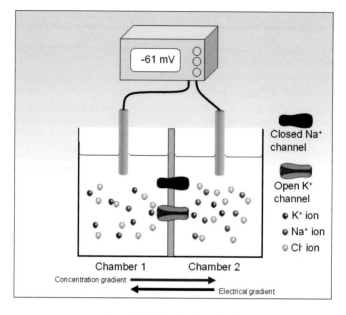

Figure 2.3. See text for details.

The potential in millivolts can be calculated using Eqn. 2.4:

$$E = 61\log\frac{[K^+]_2 + P[Na^+]_2}{[K^+]_1 + P[Na^+]_1} \tag{2.4}$$

where P is the permeability ratio, which in this case is 0.33 since Na^+ is a third less permeable than K^+. If chamber 1 represents the inside of the cell and chamber 2 the outside of the cell (usually denoted with subscripts "i" and "o" respectively) inserting the values in Table 2.1 into Eqn. 2.4 yields a membrane potential (E_m) of –23 mV. Each ion therefore experiences a different "driving force" at rest, which depends on the difference between E_m and E_{ion}. In this case there is a strong driving force (or net potential difference) for Na^+ ions to move into the cell (–23 – 61 = –84 mV) and a weaker driving force on K^+ ions (–23 – (–61) = +38 mV) causing them to move out of the cell.

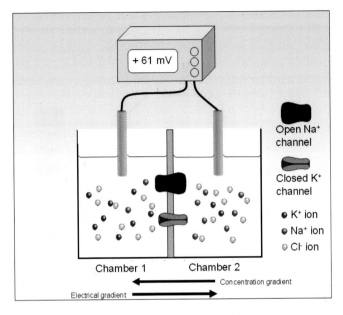

Figure 2.4. See text for details.

2.3.2.1 *What is the Goldman–Hodgkin–Katz equation?*

The plasma membrane of a real heart cell is permeable to a number of ions to greater and lesser extents. After considering the above, a better estimate of the membrane potential can be calculated by applying Eqn. 2.4. This is an abbreviated form of the Goldman–Hodgkin–Katz (GHK) equation that takes into account the relative permeabilities of the membrane to all the relevant ionic species. The equation arose initially from work published in 1943 by David Goldman of Columbia University and was derived in its current form by Nobel laureates Alan Hodgkin (Nobel Prize in Medicine in 1963) and Bernard Katz (Nobel Prize in Medicine in 1970) in a paper published in 1949 investigating the influence of the external Na^+ ion concentration on the size of the action potential. At that time they were certain that the nerve membrane changed its relative permeability to Na^+ to produce the action potential and the use of the Goldman approach allowed them to marry theoretical predictions of permeability changes with their actual measured values.

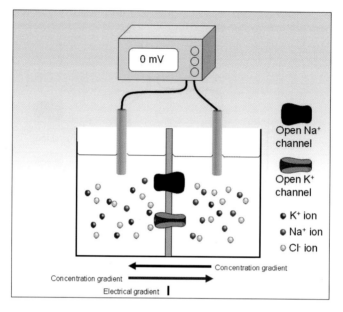

Figure 2.5. Each ion diffuses according to its concentration difference (Na^+ ion movement indicated by the blue arrow and K^+ ion movement indicated by the red arrow) and the resultant membrane potential is not at either equilibrium potential but is at 0 mV, half-way between the two equilibrium potentials.

Goldman (and also Hodgkin and Katz) assumed that the voltage gradient across the membrane was constant and that ionic movement was only influenced by diffusion and the electric field. If the permeability of a specific ion is zero, it will have no effect in determining the membrane potential. To determine membrane potential more accurately when the various ion concentrations and their relative permeabilities are known, the full GHK equation can be solved. For a membrane permeable to sodium, potassium, chloride and any ion X, the full GHK equation can be expressed as follows:

$$E = \frac{RT}{F} \ln \frac{P_K[K^+]_o + P_{Na}[Na^+]_o + P_{Cl}[Cl^-]_i + P_X[X]_o}{P_K[K^+]_i + P_{Na}[Na^+]_i + P_{Cl}[Cl^-]_o + P_X[X]_i} \qquad (2.5)$$

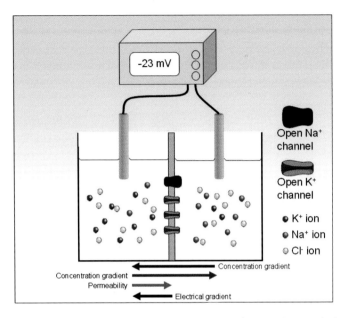

Figure 2.6. In this set-up there are three times as many K^+ channels as Na^+ channels so the membrane is much more permeable to K^+. (Na^+ ion movement is indicated by the blue arrow and K^+ ion movement is indicated by the red arrow). The final membrane potential that will be achieved at equilibrium can be calculated by taking into account the concentrations of the ions and their relative permeabilities (Eqn. 2.4).

2.3.3 What is the influence of the Na^+/K^+ pump on the membrane potential?

Recall that the resting membrane potential of a heart cell is about −80 mV, which is less negative than the equilibrium potential of K^+ ($E_K \approx -90$ mV) and so K^+ tends to move out of the cell, as the electrical potential is not sufficiently negative to match the outward concentration gradient. In addition, at −80 mV, Na^+ will tend to move into the cell, driven by both a chemical and an electrical gradient though its membrane permeability is low at rest. The steady inward leak of Na^+ and outward leak of K^+ would eventually result in the elimination of their concentration gradients, which would abolish the membrane potential.

How many ions move to produce a typical ventricular cell membrane potential?

The cell membrane can be considered to be a capacitor inasmuch as the lipid bilayer separates two chambers – intracellular and extracellular spaces – holding conducting solutions. In essence the cell membrane separates charge. Typically, cell membranes have a specific capacitance of about 1 $\mu F.cm^{-2}$ and a cardiac ventricular myocyte has dimensions approximating a box of 100 $\mu m \times 20$ $\mu m \times 10$ μm. This box therefore has a surface area of 6.4×10^{-5} cm^2 and a capacitance of ~6.4×10^{-11} F.

Now suppose that the membrane potential is –75 mV, then the charge on the membrane capacitance (Q) = V × C so:
$$Q = (75 \times 10^{-3}) \times (6.4 \times 10^{-11}) = 4.8 \times 10^{-12} \text{ C.}$$

Since the charge of an ion is 1.60×10^{-19} C then the number of ions that move is 30×10^6 or 30 million ions. This might seem a large number but such a loss has a negligible effect on the concentration gradient.

Consider that our typical ventricular myocyte of 100 $\mu m \times 20$ $\mu m \times 10$ μm has a volume of 20×10^3 μm^3. Since 1 μm^3 = 1 femtolitre (1×10^{-15} l), the cell has a volume of 20 000 fl or 20 pl.

If our cell has an intracellular $[K^+]$ = 140 mM then it contains 2.8×10^{-12} moles of K^+ ions. Remember that 1 mole corresponds to Avogadro's number of molecules (6.022×10^{23} molecules.mol^{-1}) so the cell contains 1.68×10^{12} K^+ ions.

Therefore, a loss of 30 million K^+ ions represents 0.000017% of the total number of K^+ ions.

To counteract the leak of Na^+ and K^+ and to maintain the concentration gradients upon which the membrane potential depends, the sarcolemmal Na^+/K^+ pump continually transports Na^+ out of the cell and K^+ into the cell. As the pump moves the ions against their concentration gradients, metabolic energy is required in the form of ATP hydrolysis; indeed the pump is itself an ATPase and is also referred to as the Na^+/K^+ ATPase.

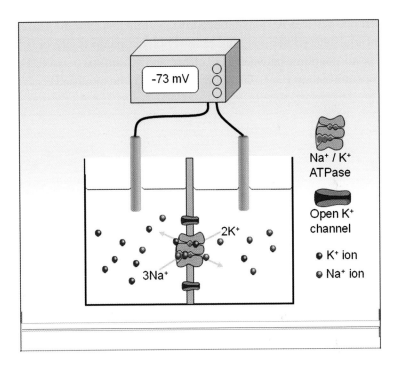

Figure 2.7. In this set-up the membrane is permeable to K^+ ions and has Na^+/K^+ pumps present. The pumps extrude three Na^+ ions for every two K^+ ions brought into the cell and are therefore electrogenic. The coupled movement of Na^+ and K^+ results in the net transfer of one positive charge out of the cell per pump cycle and this makes the membrane potential more negative that it would otherwise be if there was no electrogenic pumping.

The transfer of Na^+ and K^+ does not occur in a one-for-one electroneutral manner. The pump extrudes three Na^+ ions for every two K^+ ions brought into the cell (see Fig. 2.7). It is therefore *electrogenic* in that the net result of the coupled movement of Na^+ and K^+ is the transfer of one positive charge out of the cell, and this makes the membrane potential more negative that it would otherwise be if no electrogenic pumping existed. We can make some quantitative assessment of how much the pump activity contributes to the membrane potential by modifying Eqn. 2.4 in the same way as did Mullins and Noda in 1963. We assume that the stoichiometry of the pump is 3:2 (three Na^+ ions pumped out per two K^+ ions pumped in), and the Na^+ and K^+ fluxes are in a steady state so the coupling ratio (r) of the pump is 3/2 or 1.5. If there is no coupling between Na^+ efflux and K^+ influx, $r = 0$. For an electroneutral pump $r = 1$. Therefore Eqn. 2.4 can be modified:

$$E = 61\log\frac{r[K^+]_o + P[Na^+]_o}{r[K^+]_i + P[Na^+]_i} \qquad (2.6)$$

Using this equation and the values in Table 2.1 we can calculate that E_m is -73 mV when the pumps are present.

$$E_m = 61\log\frac{(1.5\times4)+(0.04\times140)}{(1.5\times120)+(0.04\times10)} = 61\times(-1.19) = -73\text{mV} \qquad (2.7)$$

When the pump component is removed from Eqn. 2.6 but the concentrations and relative permeabilities of the ions remain the same, then it returns to Eqn. 2.4 and using that we can calculate that E_m would be -67 mV:

$$E_m = 61\log\frac{4+(0.04\times140)}{120+(0.04\times10)} = 61\times(-1.09) = -67\text{mV} \qquad (2.8)$$

The Na^+/K^+ pump therefore contributes about 6 mV towards a negative membrane potential. It is the concentration gradient and permeability of K^+ that play the major role in the generation of the resting membrane potential. However, although the action of the Na^+/K^+ pump contributes a relatively small voltage to the formation of the total membrane potential, it is crucial to its stability because it balances the leakage of Na^+ and K^+ into and out of the cell.

2.3.4 *What is the effect of changing extracellular [K⁺] on the membrane potential?*

In the foregoing discussion we have considered idealized situations and these show that the membrane potential corresponds very closely to the predicted values of E_K (although it is slightly less negative due to a finite permeability of the membrane to other ions, notably Na$^+$) when the external K$^+$ concentration is experimentally varied. However, this only holds true when the extracellular K$^+$ concentration is above about 5 mM. In conditions of hypokalaemia, there is a marked deviation of the measured membrane potential from that calculated by the Nernst equation for K$^+$ because hypokalaemia reduces potassium *permeability*. This results in a greater influence of Na$^+$ on the membrane potential that accounts for the shift in membrane potential away from that predicted by the Nernst equation for K$^+$. This effect will be discussed in more detail in Chapter 7.

2.4 Summary

- Each ion has its own equilibrium potential.
- The resting membrane potential (E_m) is a compromise between various E_{ion} weighted by concentration and permeability.
- The membrane potential is described by the GHK equation.
- Resting E_m is usually dominated by K$^+$ ions.
- There will be a flux across the membrane for any ion where $E_m \neq E_{ion}$.
- If E_m is stable then net flow of ionic charge is zero.

2.5 Questions

Using the values in Table 2.1:
(1)   Calculate the E_m of a cell at rest assuming an active Na$^+$/K$^+$ pump with a stoichiometry of 3:2.

(2)   At the peak of an action potential the relative permeabilities of ions through a membrane change to $P_K:P_{Na}:P_{Cl}$ =1:15:0.1. Calculate E_m assuming no contribution of the Na$^+$/K$^+$ pump.

(3)   If the external K$^+$ concentration is increased by a factor of 10, what is the new value of E_K?

2.6 Bibliography

Goldman, D.E. (1943). Potential, impedance and rectification in membranes. *J. Gen. Physiol.* **27**, 37–60.

Hodgkin, A.L. and Katz, B. (1949). The effect of sodium ions on the electrical activity of the giant axon of the squid. *J. Physiol.* **108**, 37–77.

Mullins, L.J. and Noda, K. (1963). The influence of sodium-free solutions on the membrane potential of frog muscle fibers. *J. Gen. Physiol.* **47**, 117–132.

Chapter 3

Measuring Membrane Currents

In August 1939 Alan Hodgkin and Andrew Huxley began a series of experiments to elucidate the time course of membrane permeability changes to sodium and potassium ions that underlie the nerve action potential. Although carried out in the nerve, the work of Hodgkin and Huxley is fundamental for an understanding of trans-membrane events that occur during the cardiac action potential. World War II halted their work, but they continued after the war and in 1952 published a series of papers that developed a mathematical model of a nerve action potential which explained their experimental observations. In 1963 Hodgkin and Huxley won the Nobel Prize in Physiology and Medicine for that work and they received knighthoods in 1972 and 1974 respectively.

3.1 Chapter objectives

After reading this chapter you should be able to:

- Understand the elementary concepts of electricity as applied to excitable cells
- Describe the early experiments of Hodgkin and Huxley
- Plot and perform simple analyses of current–voltage relationships from voltage clamp experiments
- Explain what the experiments of Hodgkin and Huxley suggest about channel gating
- Explain the reason for the phenomenon of refractory period

3.2 Key electrical concepts: voltage, current, conductance and capacitance

There are a number of concepts that are important to understand when talking about membrane currents.

3.2.1 *Voltage*

We introduced the concept of voltage (V) in the previous chapter when describing how a potential difference (or membrane potential, E_m) is formed across a heart cell membrane. Work is needed to move a charged species through a potential difference and, conversely, energy is released when a charged species moves from a point with higher potential to a point of lower potential. One joule (J) of work is needed to move one coulomb (C) of charge (Q) through a potential difference of one volt. One volt is equivalent to 1 J.C^{-1}.

Most voltages we will deal with are of the order of millivolts, though in biology there are examples of animals being able to produce very large voltages. The electric eel (*Electrophorus electricus*) is named because of the large electrical discharge it can produce to stun prey and deter predators. Its tail contains specialized cells called electrocytes that generate voltages and store energy like a biological battery. When it is threatened or is attacking prey, these cells discharge simultaneously, often producing between 400 and 600 volts.

3.2.2 *Current*

Current is denoted by the symbol I and is measured in amperes or amps (A). One ampere is the flow of one coulomb of charge past a point in one second. Most currents flowing through the membranes of heart cells are of the order of nanoamps and currents flowing through single channels are of picoamps in magnitude. In reality, even though electrons flow from a more negative point to a more positive point, we say that current flows from positive to negative, i.e. in the opposite direction. This is purely convention. The size of the current (I) flowing through a conductor is proportional to the voltage across the conductor and its conductance (G):

$$I = G \times V \qquad (3.1)$$

3.2.3 Conductance

The conductance depends on the concentration of the charged species, their mobility and the conductor's geometry. Generally, conductance increases when the density and mobility of charged species increase. It is helpful for electrophysiologists to think of conductance rather than resistance. A small resistance is a large conductance, since conductance is the reciprocal of resistance:

$$G = \frac{1}{R} \qquad (3.2)$$

The unit of conductance is the siemens (S). The unit of resistance (R) is the ohm (Ω).

Equation 3.1 is simply a form of Ohm's law ($I = V/R$), but expressed in terms of conductance and not resistance. Conductance of a membrane is related to its permeability in the sense that the amount of charged species and how fast they each move across the membrane depends on how permeable it is to the particular species. However, conductance and permeability are not the same (see Table 3.1).

Conductance depends on	*Permeability* depends on
Membrane potential	Membrane potential
Type of ion	Type of ion
Concentration of ion	

Table 3.1

Recall from Chapter 2 that the driving force (i.e. the voltage) on an ion is ($E_m - E_{ion}$). Therefore we can apply Ohm's law or Eqn. 3.1, and so the current we can measure flowing through a membrane is given by:

$$I = G \times (E_m - E_{ion})$$ (3.3)

3.2.4 *Capacitance*

The slightly tricky electrical quantity to understand is capacitance.   If two conductors are separated by an insulator it is possible to generate a potential difference between them by moving charge from one conductor to the other. The voltage between the conductors is proportional to the charge moved so:

$$V = k \times Q$$ (3.4)

where k is a constant that depends on the size of the conductors and the type of insulator.   The reciprocal of this constant k is called the capacitance (C) and has units of coulomb.volt^{-1} or farad (F). Therefore:

$$C = \frac{Q}{V}$$ (3.5)

A capacitor of 1 farad with 1 volt across its conductors has +1 coulomb of stored charge on one conductor and −1 coulomb on the other. Whereas the current flowing through a resistor is proportional to the voltage across the resistor, the current flowing through a circuit containing a capacitor is proportional to the *rate of change of voltage*. So if you wish to change the voltage across a farad by one volt per second, you have to supply one amp of current to do so. A farad is quite a large quantity, particularly when used in electrophysiological discussions of single excitable cells. A heart cell membrane has about 70–200 pF of capacitance. The current flowing in a capacitor during charging is:

$$I = C \frac{\delta V}{\delta t}$$ (3.6)

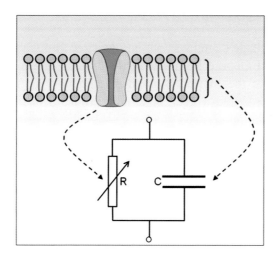

Figure 3.1. The lipid bilayer constitutes the membrane capacitance and the ion channels are the equivalent of variable conductors (or resistors) connected in parallel across the cell membrane.

To appreciate the importance of the quantity of capacitance we have to realize that the electrical equivalent of the cell membrane, which comprises a lipid bilayer and ion transport proteins, is approximately as shown in Fig. 3.1. The bilayer constitutes the membrane capacitance and the ion channels are the equivalent of variable conductors (or resistors) connected in parallel across the cell membrane. With this simplified arrangement the total current (I_m) flowing across the membrane is:

$$I_m = I_i \times C \frac{\delta V}{\delta t} \tag{3.7}$$

where I_i is the component of current that flows through the various ion transport mechanisms. The main problem with trying to measure I_m is that the capacitive current is large and flows rapidly, so it can overlap and therefore mask I_i. The solution to this problem is to *"voltage clamp"* the preparation and measure current when voltage is not changing. In this way the capacitive element of the total membrane current can be ignored.

3.3 What is voltage clamp?

The concept of voltage clamp was put into practice through the efforts of Kenneth Cole and George Marmont in the 1940s. They shared some laboratory space at the Marine Biological Laboratory in Woods Hole, Massachusetts, USA, and worked on similar problems of trying to keep the membrane potential of a cell at a level set by the experimenter and to record the ionic current needed to hold this potential. They apparently never got on very well, but their individual methods were melded together later by Alan Hodgkin, Andrew Huxley and Bernard Katz to produce an elegant and effective device using two electrodes that could adequately control (or clamp) the membrane potential of a squid nerve cell at any voltage desired by the experimenter. A fascinating account of how Hodgkin, Huxley and Katz came together to work on the ionic basis of the nerve action potential is given by Hodgkin himself in a Review Lecture delivered to the Centenary Meeting of the Physiological Society in Cambridge, UK, in July 1976.

Many early voltage clamp experiments were carried out using the large nerve cells dissected from squid (*Loligo pealeii* or *forbesii*). The axons of the nerves that innervate the mantle of the squid are some of the largest in nature (up to 1 mm in diameter and up to 10 cm in length). These nerves control parts of the squid's water jet propulsion system which creates very rapid movements through the water. Their large diameters allow experimenters to insert low resistance electrodes into their lumens with relative ease and to perfuse them internally with solutions containing known concentrations of important ions. Using large axial electrodes enables the experimenters to clamp the axon quickly to a particular voltage and ensures that most of the axon is at the same potential.

The membrane potential is measured with an electrode placed inside and along the long axis of the axon (Fig. 3.2). This electrode is connected to an amplifier that compares the voltage inside the cell with an external reference electrode. The measurement of membrane potential is fed to another amplifier that compares it (E_m) with the voltage that the experimenter has set – termed the command voltage (E_c).

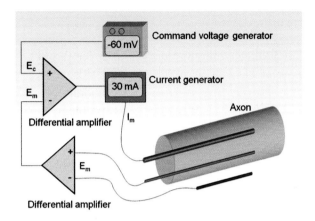

Figure 3 .2. A simplification of a voltage clamp set-up.

The output of this amplifier is fed back into the axon via a second electrode. This feedback circuit is designed to hold the membrane potential at the desired value even when the permeability of the membrane changes during an excitatory event. If the E_m is different from the E_c, current is injected into the axon via the current electrode to cause the E_m to become the same as E_c. The current that flows into the axon to keep the membrane at the desired E_c can be measured and equals (but is opposite to) the amount of current flowing across the active nerve membrane. By keeping the membrane potential constant, ionic currents can be measured that will reflect the conductance of the membrane at that specific voltage, thereby giving us insight into how the membrane potential influences the permeability properties of ion channels and thus how it influences ionic current flow across the membrane.

From information derived from their voltage clamp experiments, Hodgkin and Huxley developed their model of action potential generation for which they subsequently were awarded the Nobel Prize in 1963. We will review some of the key experiments of their work because these remain, even now, essential for the understanding of action potential generation in all excitable cells. The voltage clamp method is still widely used to study ionic currents in many cell types, although it has been refined (particularly in the form of the patch clamp technique).

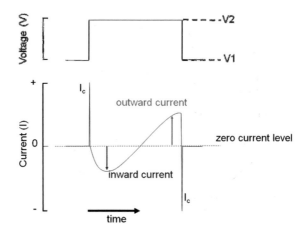

Figure 3.3.   Typical voltage clamp traces. Large, but brief, capacitive currents (I_c) are seen when the voltage changes from V1 to V2, such as moving from the resting membrane potential to a new desired potential and vice versa, but are eliminated once the voltage is kept constant, during which time the magnitude and direction of ionic currents can be studied.

The patch clamp variation has adequate resolution to measure the current flowing through a single ion channel. Some voltage clamp conventions, as seen in Fig. 3.3, include:
- Inward current: positively charged ions moving into cell, seen as a downward deflection on a current trace (though in Hodgkin and Huxley's original papers inward current was upward)
- Inward current depolarizes a cell under voltage clamp
- Depolarization means that the cell interior becomes more positive
- Hyperpolarization means that the cell interior becomes more negative

A typical example of a voltage clamp experiment done by Hodgkin and Huxley is shown in Fig. 3.3. The membrane potential is initially clamped at the voltage V1 and then changed to V2. Large but very brief capacitance currents flow during the voltage changes. The current recording shows inward current flow followed by outward flow.

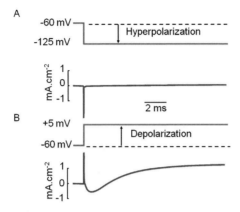

Figure 3.4. Panel A shows current evoked by a clamp step from –60 to –125 mV. The very rapid and unresolvable downstroke at the beginning of the current trace is the capacitive current flowing during the voltage change. Following the capacitive current change no other current flows while the membrane is held at –125 mV. Panel B shows the current evoked following the same size of voltage step in the positive direction from –60 mV to +5 mV. The membrane is charged by the voltage step eliciting capacitive current, but then this is followed within 1 ms by an inward current which, in turn, develops into a more slowly increasing or delayed outward current that reaches a maximum around 10 ms.

3.4 Hodgkin and Huxley experiments

One of the first voltage clamp experiments by Hodgkin and Huxley is shown in Fig. 3.4. Panel A shows current that is evoked following a clamp step of –65 mV from a resting E_m of –60 mV, i.e. a step to a potential of –125 mV. (In their initial studies Hodgkin and Huxley could not measure the absolute membrane potential but instead recorded changes in membrane potential from a "resting" value. From their recordings of action potentials it is generally assumed that they used axons that had resting membrane potentials on average around –60 mV). The very rapid and un-resolvable upstroke is the capacitive current flowing essentially during the voltage change. This current flow is over within 23–30 μs and, although large, is too rapid for its time course to be recorded faithfully. Following the capacitive current the trace is "flat", indicating that there is no other current flowing while the membrane is hyperpolarized at this potential. On the other hand, Panel B shows the current evoked following a similar sized voltage step but this time in the positive or depolarizing direction from –60 mV to +5 mV. Again, the membrane is charged by the voltage step eliciting capacitive current but then this is followed within 1 ms by an inward current. This, in turn, develops into a more slowly increasing or delayed outward current that reaches a maximum around 10 ms from the start of the clamp step.

This experiment clearly demonstrates that the size and direction of current flow through the membrane is voltage dependent. Notice that Hodgkin and Huxley calibrated their records in terms of *current density*. Current density is the amount of current passing through a cross-sectional area of a conductor in a given time. This calibration is crucial because larger cells produce more current, so one way of normalising the results is to express the values in terms of an area of axon membrane – cm^2. Nowadays we tend to express current density in terms of the capacitance of the cell since this is directly proportional to its surface area and thus size.

Hodgkin and Huxley then investigated how the properties of the early inward and late outward currents changed as the membrane potential was varied over a larger voltage range. Typical results of these experiments are shown in Fig. 3.5. The traces have had the very fast capacitance current component removed. In Panel A, as the depolarizations or clamp steps become more positive (than about –55 mV), the direction of current flow is initially inward then outward. The early current (measured about 1 ms after the depolarizing step, as shown in Panel B) becomes larger following increasing depolarization but then as the clamp steps become more positive this component of current decreases in size. The late current (which Hodgkin and Huxley measured about 8 ms after the depolarizing step, as shown in Panel B) increases with increasing depolarization and continues to do so even following very positive clamp steps. If we measure the maximum inward currents at a fixed time following the clamp steps and plot these against the voltage to which the axon is depolarized, we generate a so-called *current–voltage (I–V)* relationship shown (by the filled squares, ■) in panel C.

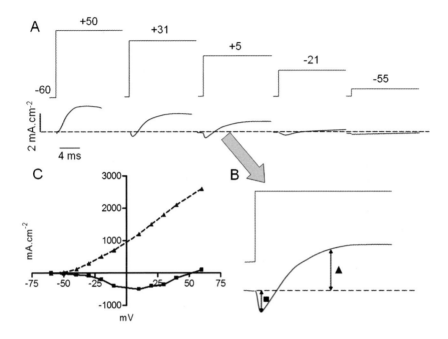

Figure 3.5. Panel A shows a series of voltage clamp steps (red) that produce inward and outward currents (blue). Using the current trace produced by the clamp step to +5 mV as an example (Panel B), inward and outward currents are measured as indicated by the filled square (■) and filled triangle (▲) respectively. These currents are then plotted on the graph (Panel C) that illustrates the *I–V* relationships of early and late currents.

Following very positive steps, the graph shows that the early current reverses in polarity around +55 mV, which is near to the Na$^+$ equilibrium potential. In these experiments, the seawater bathing the axons had a Na$^+$ concentration of about 440 mM and the intra-axon Na$^+$ concentration was about 50 mM, so E_{Na} would be +57 mV.

We can also measure the size of the outward currents at a fixed time following the clamp step and plot these against the voltage (the filled triangles, ▲). Notice that at potentials more negative than about –50 mV the current through the membrane is very low, but at more positive potentials the late currents are greatly increased in size. The *I–V* relationship of these late currents is not linear (at some voltages no current flows at all and at others a large amount of current flows) and demonstrates the phenomenon of *delayed rectification*. The term "rectification" is used to describe the non-linear nature of current flow in an analogous way to an electrical rectifier (see also Chapter 7, pp. 183–198). The term "delayed" refers to the outward current that flows later than the early inward current, i.e. it is delayed in time.

3.4.1 *Separating the early and late currents*

The fact that the early current flow reverses in polarity at essentially the same voltage as the calculated Na^+ equilibrium potential suggests that the early inward current is carried by Na^+ moving into the axon. Hodgkin and Huxley devised an unequivocal way of testing this suggestion by carrying out the same voltage clamp experiment but in the absence of extracellular Na^+. To maintain tonicity of the extracellular solution, they substituted the Na^+ in the artificial sea water by choline, an organic compound that would not flow across the axon membrane. The traces from such a series of experiments are shown in Fig. 3.6.

In normal sea water the currents evoked on various depolarizations have the same form as before, but when Na^+ is removed from the sea water the early inward currents do not appear – there are only outwardly moving late currents (Fig. 3.6 Panel A). This experiment demonstrates that the early inward current must be due to Na^+ entering the axon. The removal of Na^+ did not affect the form of the late outward current so this suggested to Hodgkin and Huxley that this current must be due to a different ion, the most likely being K^+. To illustrate the time course of the flow of the Na^+ current (I_{Na}) following depolarization, they subtracted the current obtained in the absence of Na^+ from that obtained in the presence of the ion for each clamp step (Fig. 3.6 Panel B). The subtracted current showed the form of the current carried by Na^+ alone. The traces of the currents recorded in normal sea water ($I_{Na} + I_K$) and that recorded in Na^+-free artificial sea water (I_K) could be superimposed at later times, so this suggested to Hodgkin and Huxley that the late outward currents were carried by K^+. Therefore, following a depolarization of the membrane from E_m there is an early influx of Na^+ into the cell – producing a transient inward current – followed by a delayed efflux of

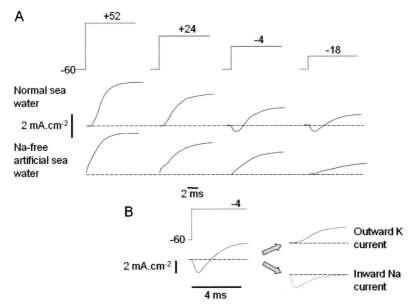

Figure 3.6. In normal sea water the currents evoked by various depolarizations follow a similar pattern to those in Fig. 3.5. When Na⁺ is removed from the sea water, the early inward currents disappear.

K⁺ from the cell – producing a sustained outward current. It appears that Na⁺ channels first become conductive then "switch off"; K⁺ channels become conductive more slowly and remain so until the cell is repolarized.

3.4.2 *Na⁺ and K⁺ channels conduct in a voltage- and time-dependent manner*

Hodgkin and Huxley found that they could describe these changes in ionic conductances by using Eqn. 3.4:

$$G_{\text{Na}} = \frac{I_{\text{Na}}}{(E - E_{\text{Na}})}$$

(3.8)

$$G_K = \frac{I_K}{(E - E_K)} \qquad (3.9)$$

When they calculated G_{Na} and G_K (now both positive quantities) following various clamp steps they found that they were both voltage and time dependent (Fig. 3.7). By time dependent we mean that the conductances (i.e. ion channels) take some time to "switch on" or activate. They do so at different speeds, with the Na^+ conductance reaching a maximum more rapidly than the more slowly activating K^+ conductance. The other difference is that the Na^+ conductance also "switches off" or inactivates rapidly even though the membrane potential is kept at a depolarized level, in contrast to the K^+ conductance which does not appear to inactivate. By voltage dependent we mean two things. Firstly, the speed of the activation and (for the Na^+ conductance) inactivation increases as the size of the depolarizing clamp step increases. Secondly, both conductances increase as the size of the depolarizing clamp step increases. We will look more closely at the processes of activation and inactivation in the next section and take this a stage further in order to understand the mechanism that allows the conductances to sense the voltage changes across the membrane.

3.4.3 *Activation and inactivation of channels*

Clearly Hodgkin and Huxley did not know the nature of these conductance mechanisms, but they were fairly sure that nerves and other excitable cells had pores or channels within their plasma membranes that allowed ions to pass quite selectively (since ion substitution experiments showed different results) from one side to the other. They were beginning to understand that these channels opened and closed (so conducted or not) in response to the voltage across the membrane.

The time course of the increase in K^+ channel conductance or activation is slightly easier to express in the form of an equation than the Na^+ conductance changes, so we will introduce the concepts involved with reference to this (see Figs. 3.7 and 3.8).

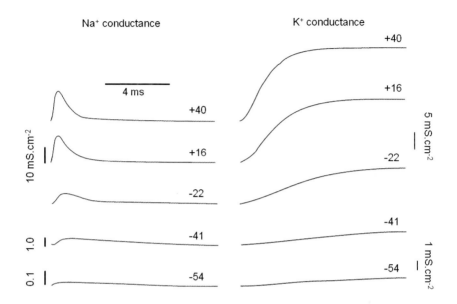

Figure 3.7. The voltage and time dependency of Na$^+$ and K$^+$ conductance changes. Note the variations in scaling on some traces. The conductance changes have been evoked using the voltage clamp steps (in mV) shown.

Following a depolarization there is a slow increase in conductance that has an approximate sigmoidal shape over time. Following repolarization, the K$^+$ conductance declines rather more exponentially (Fig. 3.8).

Hodgkin and Huxley found an equation that fitted the observed conductance changes with reasonable accuracy. In their 1952 paper they discussed that a sigmoid curve would result from co-operative processes with several (first order) reactions occurring simultaneously. The shape of the curve depends on the number of reactions, and the greater the number, the more pronounced the inflexion of the curve.

The shape of the experimentally measured increase in conductance was best fitted by a variable (which they called, *n*) raised to the power of 4. This variable has no dimensions and simply has a value between 0

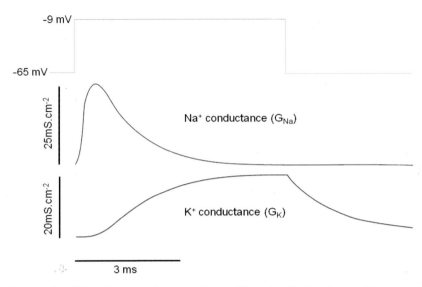

Figure 3.8.   Following a depolarization from –65 to –9 mV, there is a rapid increase in Na$^+$ conductance which then declines rapidly. During the depolarization there is a slow increase in K$^+$ conductance which has an approximate sigmoidal shape. Following repolarization, the K$^+$ conductance declines more exponentially.

and 1 as a function of voltage and time. Hodgkin and Huxley surmised that the channels contained several particles (or gates), all of which had to be in appropriate position (or open) at once in order for the channel to conduct. This co-operative mechanism gave rise to the sigmoid shape of the conductance curve.

The rather neat consequence of this notion was that if only one particle, or "*gate*", was out of position, then the channel itself shut, so producing the exponential fall in the conductance curve. One could envisage each channel either being composed of four individual particles or as a pore with four gates lined up sequentially inside. In order for the channel to be open and allow ions to flow through, all the particles or gates must be lined up or open simultaneously. If one particle or gate is out of alignment or closed then the channel cannot conduct the ion.

Using Eqn. 3.3, the maximum K$^+$ current produced from the conductance change at any given time can now be represented by:

$$I_K = n^4 \overline{G_K}(E - E_K) \tag{3.10}$$

where $\overline{G_K}$ represents the maximum K$^+$ conductance and n^4 represents the probability that all four particles are in an open or conducting configuration.

The individual particles or gates move into position to open and close the channel randomly but rapidly. The key point to understand is that the probability that any one gating particle confers an open position for the channel is dependent on the voltage across the membrane. The particles are charged, so the position they occupy within the membrane is affected by the electrical potential across the membrane, and this determines whether the channel with which they are associated is open or closed – hence they are voltage gated. Following depolarization of the membrane, there will be a greater probability that the particles will be in the correct position for the channel to be open. We can take this line of thinking a stage further.

The random motion of channel particles (Brownian motion is an example) means that the transition between closed and open conformations of a pore is a random event. It is not possible to predict whether any channel will be open or closed at any time, but we can, using laws of probability, assess if a channel is more or less likely to behave in a particular way. Hence, as the extent of depolarization is increased, it is more likely that K$^+$ channels will be in an open conformation and for longer periods. It is apparent that the kinetic features of each single channel are important in determining the characteristics of the whole (cell) K$^+$ current.

The changes in Na$^+$ channel conductance are more difficult to model. This is because the sodium conductance shows both activation and inactivation. The inactivation process – like that of activation – is also a function of voltage and time (see Info Box on p. 55). The increase and decrease of Na^+ channel conductance can be best described using the product of two variables, an activation parameter termed m and an inactivation parameter termed h. Like the n variable, they both can vary in value from 0 to 1. Again, using Eqn. 3.3, the maximum Na^+ current produced from the changes in conductance could be calculated by solving the following:

$$I_{Na} = m^3 h \overline{G_{Na}} (E - E_{Na}) \qquad (3.11)$$

Where $\overline{G_{Na}}$ is the maximum Na^+ conductance; m^3 represents the probability that all three activation particles are in the open configuration and the inactivation parameter h represents the probability that the Na^+ channel is not inactivated. In an analogous way to K^+ channels, Hodgkin and Huxley proposed that each Na^+ channel contains three activation particles or gates (m particles) which respond rapidly to a trans-membrane voltage change, and one inactivation particle or gate (h particle) which reacts to a voltage change more slowly. They envisaged the processes of activation and inactivation involving the sequential movement of these particles (Fig. 3.9).

At the resting potential, the h particle is in a position to allow the channel to conduct, but the m particles are positioned such that the channel is closed and cannot conduct. When the membrane is depolarized from the resting potential, the m particles sense the voltage change, move accordingly, and the channel opens or activates. After a short time the h particle moves into a different configuration and the channel closes despite the membrane still being depolarized. The channel is now in a so-called inactivated state. If the membrane is now repolarized, the m and h particles reconfigure to form a closed state. Once the channel returns to a closed state it can be opened again in response to depolarization. Inactivated Na^+ channels cannot be reactivated to their conducting state directly – the inactivation must be removed by repolarizing the membrane. If the membrane is depolarized during the time of inactivation the channel remains closed in its inactivated state. This is the mechanism that underlies the absolute refractory period of an action potential (see Chapter 6).

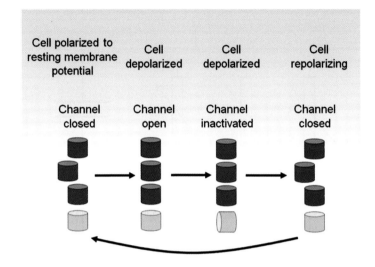

Figure 3.9. At the resting potential, the *h* particle is in a position to allow the channel to conduct, but the *m* particles are positioned so that the Na$^+$ channel cannot conduct. It is in a closed state. If the membrane is depolarized, the *m* particles respond and form an open conformation. The channel is in an activated state and conducts. After a short time the *h* particle moves to close the channel despite the membrane still being depolarized. The channel is now in an inactivated state. It will not return to a closed state until the membrane is repolarized.

3.5 Conclusions

The electrical equivalent of the membrane can be imagined to be similar to that shown in Fig. 3.10, with parallel conductances that vary and the currents driven by the electrochemical gradient (the batteries). There is also a leak conductance to account for some small current that flowed all the time. Hodgkin and Huxley's voltage clamp experiments and their mathematical analyses and treatment of these experiments allowed them to account for the different time courses and voltage dependencies of Na$^+$ and K$^+$ channels during the action potential.

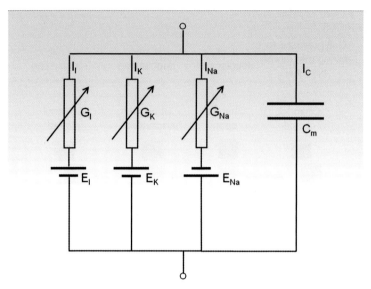

Figure 3.10.   An electrical analogy of a membrane of an excitable cell. The capacitance is the electrical equivalent of the lipid bilayer. In parallel are various pathways for ionic flow which vary in conductance. The currents are driven by the electrochemical gradient (the batteries). There is also a leak conductance (G_l) to account for some small current that flows all the time.

In fact, using the equations alone they were able to reconstruct the shape of the membrane voltage changes during the action potential and make predictions on how the axon would respond to stimuli of varying intensity. Their views that the channels could be open or closed depending on the conformation of certain molecules provided a working framework for the development of a large number of experiments and models of ion conduction and action potential production in other excitable cells. Although there are flaws in some of their arguments, the papers set a precedent and focused thinking on how ion channels worked.

Ions cross membranes through channels that are either in an open or closed state. A channel will be in an open state if all the voltage sensor particles of the channel are in an open configuration. The total current in the cell flowing through a particular population of channels will be the sum of the current flowing through the individual channels in the open state.

Inactivation of Na$^+$ conductance is also time and voltage dependent

Depolarization has two effects on the Na$^+$ conductance. Initially, there is activation of the ion channel and current flow increases. This is followed by inactivation which turns off the current flow. Experiments showing that this latter process is voltage and time dependent are shown in Fig. 3.11.

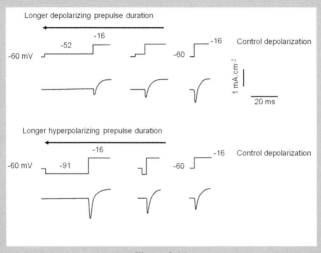

Figure 3.11

The normal current elicited from a control clamp step is shown on the top trace. The clamp step is a depolarization from −60 to −16 mV. The test protocols always include this control but interpose a very small depolarizing clamp step to −52 mV, which progressively increases in time. As the length of the prepulse is increased, the inward Na$^+$ current activated by the main step becomes smaller and smaller. The implication from such an experiment is that the small depolarization inactivates some Na$^+$ channels. The longer the membrane is held at this slightly depolarized level, the larger the Na$^+$ inactivation. In other words, the inactivation process is time dependent.

The process of Na$^+$ inactivation can be effectively removed by first hyperpolarizing the cell before applying the control depolarizing clamp step, as shown in the lower panel of Fig. 3.11. Progressively longer periods of hyperpolarization result in larger Na$^+$ currents elicited by the depolarizing step.

Given what we now know about how channels gate and reflecting on what experimental tools were at their disposal at the time, the work is quite extraordinary. Since the Hodgkin and Huxley work was published, the advances in electrophysiological techniques in combination with those of molecular biology and X-ray crystallography have allowed huge advances in understanding ion channel structure and function, but the ideas introduced by the Nobel winners still underpin the topic.

3.6 Summary

- Voltage clamp allows control over the membrane potential so that ionic currents can be measured. The currents reflect the conductance of the membrane at specific voltages, thereby giving insight into how the membrane potential influences the permeability properties of ion channels and thus how it influences ionic current flow across the membrane.

- Conventions for voltage clamp generally are that:
    - Inward current is observed as a downward deflection on a current trace
    - Inward current depolarizes a cell under voltage clamp because positively charged ions move into the cell
    - Depolarization means the cell interior becomes more positive
    - Hyperpolarization means the cell interior becomes more negative

- Early voltage clamp experiments on squid giant axons showed that, following a depolarization of the membrane, there is an early influx of Na^+ ions into the cell – producing a transient inward current – followed by a delayed efflux of K^+ ions from the cell – producing a sustained outward current. Na^+ channels first become conductive then "switch off" or inactivate, and K^+ channels become conductive more slowly and remain so until the cell is repolarized.

Na⁺ channel inactivation is voltage dependent

The experiment in Fig. 3.12 uses long conditioning pulses so that the effects of depolarization or hyperpolarization develop maximally. Large pre-depolarizations inhibit the inward current in response to the test pulses while, conversely, pre-hyperpolarization makes the inward current larger. Using measurements derived from these experiments, the graph beneath was constructed by plotting the maximum size of the inward current obtained with the control clamp step divided by that obtained by other steps against the voltage of the prepulse. This gives a picture of the voltage dependency of Na⁺ current inactivation. Hodgkin and Huxley assigned a dimensionless inactivation variable they called h, with a value of 1 when no inactivation occurred, and a value of 0 when inactivation was complete.

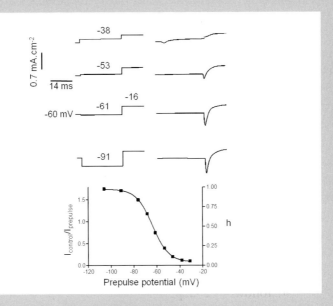

Figure 3.12

- If a channel has time-dependent behaviour, we mean that its conductance takes some time to "switch on" or activate. The conductance of Na^+ channels reaches a maximum more rapidly than K^+ channel conductances.

- If a channel is voltage dependent, its speed of activation and the size of the current it passes vary with the size of the depolarizing clamp step.

- Channel activation is governed by particles or gates that move into position to open and close the channel randomly. The probability that any one gating particle confers an open position for the channel is dependent on the voltage across the membrane. Following depolarization of the membrane, there will be a greater probability that the particles will be in the correct position for the channel to be open.

- The kinetic features of each single channel are important in determining the characteristics of the whole cell current.

- Na^+ channels show both activation and inactivation. The inactivation process is a function of voltage and time. In Na^+ channels the inactivation process takes longer to occur than activation. When channels are inactivated they remain shut despite the membrane still being depolarized. Repolarization of the membrane is required to remove the inactivation and return the channels to a closed state from which they can be activated.

3.7 Questions

(1) What is the difference between conductance and permeability?

(2) Na^+ channels show both activation and inactivation. Describe in simple Hodgkin and Huxley terms the processes of activation and inactivation.

(3) Some true/false questions to test your understanding:
- (a) Current is the flow of 1 coulomb of charge past a point in 1 second
- (b) Conductance is the reciprocal of resistance
- (c) Ohm's law is defined as $I = V/R$
- (d) The flow of Na^+ and K^+ ions through their channels is only voltage dependent
- (e) The early inward current is due to K^+
- (f) The late outward current is due to Na^+
- (g) Na^+ conductance is influenced by activation and inactivation of the ion channel

3.8 Bibliography

3.8.1 *Books and reviews*

Aidley, D.J. (1998). *The Physiology of Excitable Cells* (4th edn). Cambridge University Press.

Cole, K.S. (1982). Squid axon membrane: impedance decrease to voltage clamp. *Ann. Rev. Neurosci.* **5**, 305–323.

Hille, B. (2001). *Ion Channels of Excitable Membranes* (3rd edn). Sinauer Associates Inc.

Hodgkin, A.L. (1976). Chance and design in electrophysiology: an informal account of certain experiments on nerve carried out between 1934 and 1952. *J. Physiol.* **263**, 1–21.

Hodgkin, A.L. (1983). Beginning: some reminiscences of my early life (1914–1947). *Ann. Rev. Physiol.* **45**, 1–16.

3.8.2 *Original papers*

Hodgkin, A.L. and Katz, B. (1949). The effect of sodium ions on the electrical activity of the giant axon of the squid. *J. Physiol.* **108**, 37–77.

Hodgkin, A.L., Huxley, A.F. and Katz, B. (1952). Measurement of current–voltage relations in the membrane of the giant axon of *Loligo*. *J. Physiol.* **116**, 424–448.

Hodgkin, A.L. and Huxley, A.F. (1952). Currents carried by sodium and potassium ions through the membrane of the giant axon of *Loligo*. *J. Physiol.* **116**, 449–472.

Hodgkin, A.L. and Huxley, A.F. (1952). The dual effect of membrane potential on sodium conductance in the giant axon of *Loligo*. *J. Physiol.* **116**, 497–506.

Hodgkin, A.L. and Huxley, A.F. (1952). A quantitative description of membrane current and its application to conduction and excitation in nerve. *J. Physiol.* **117**, 500–544.

Chapter 4

Channel Structure and Function

The work of Hodgkin and Huxley summarized in Chapter 3 laid the foundations for our knowledge of ion channels, particularly in excitable cells. The channels allow ions to cross a rather inhospitable area (the hydrophobic lipid bilayer) if they are in an open configuration. Channel opening in the squid axon membrane is governed by a voltage sensor that moves according to the trans-membrane potential.

4.1 Chapter objectives

After reading this chapter you should know:
- That channels open in response to various stimuli
- That total membrane current equals the sum of small (unitary) currents flowing through individual channels
- The typical structure of voltage-gated K^+ channels
- How channels are thought to sense voltage changes across the cell membrane
- How channels discriminate between ions
- How channels are thought to inactivate

4.2 Ions flow through separate channels

The total (or macroscopic) current flowing through a particular population of channels will be the sum of the (microscopic) currents flowing through all the individual channels that are in an open state. In more mathematical terms the membrane current, I, equals the current flowing through one channel, i, times the number of open channels, N_o.

$$I = i \times N_o \qquad (4.1)$$

The predictions made by Hodgkin and Huxley (latterly in collaboration with Katz) were confirmed by Hille in the late 1960s. By then, work by Toshio Narahashi and John Moore at Duke University, using Moore's sucrose gap voltage clamp technique, established that a neurotoxin called tetrodotoxin (TTX) blocked the Na^+ conductance very specifically. In fact, TTX was so specific an inhibitor that it was (and still is) an indispensable tool in identifying individual components of membrane current. Radioactively labelled toxin is used in assessing channel density and in purifying channel preparations used for structural studies (see box below). Around the same time, Hagiwara and Armstrong discovered that tetraethylammonium (TEA) ions blocked the K^+ conductance very selectively. Hille then performed very convincing voltage clamp experiments that demonstrated axons treated with TTX only displayed delayed outward current and axons perfused with TEA only exhibited the inactivating inward current.

Experiments over the following years reached several conclusions about the properties of channels.

4.3   Channels can be activated (or "gated") in various ways

The transition between a channel's open and closed state is called "gating". It became clear that channel gating occurred in response to different stimuli and, accordingly, channels fall broadly into three categories: those that are "ligand-gated", where the opening of the channel is dictated by the presence of a substance (e.g. the acetylcholine-sensitive channel at the neuromuscular junction); those that are "voltage-gated", where the channel opens in response to a voltage across the membrane (e.g. the Na^+ channel in the giant axon); and those that respond to mechanical stimuli (e.g. stretch-sensitive Cl^- channels involved in cellular volume regulation).

4.4 Channels are specialized to allow the transport of specific ionic species

Na^+ and K^+ ions crossed cell membranes independently so, in each of the broad categories, there are channels that allowed the transport of specific ions. Key pieces of evidence that supported the existence of independent channels came from experiments using neurotoxins and TEA. The fact that TTX could eliminate the Na^+ currents when applied to the outside of the squid axon leaving K^+ currents unaffected strongly suggested that Na^+ ions pass only through specific Na^+ channels. Correspondingly, since K^+ currents could be very specifically blocked by TEA application, it seemed that there were two separate pathways for Na^+ and K^+ flux across cell membranes.

4.5 Channels can discriminate between ions

It follows logically from Section 4.2 that the different types of channel have to be capable of discriminating between Na^+, K^+ and various other ions, so allowing only one particular ionic species to flow through them given appropriate conditions.

4.6 Channels can pass large ionic currents

Channels appeared to be able to allow ions to pass through them at high rates because the macroscopic (summed) ionic currents could be large. To understand this point better we can calculate how many ions pass through a typical K^+ channel in one second. Some K^+ channels called BK (which stands for big K), Maxi-K or slo1 channels have conductances of 100 pS (picosiemens) or larger. They are activated by changes in membrane potential and by increases in the concentration of intracellular Ca^{2+}, and are thought to provide a negative feedback system to inhibit excitation induced by the opening of Ca^{2+} channels. Recall from Chapter 3 that:

$$I = G \times (E_m - E_{ion}) \qquad (4.2)$$

Tetrodotoxin

Tetrodotoxin (TTX) is found in pufferfish (*Tetraodontidae*), porcupinefish (*Diodontidae*), the blue-ringed octopus (*Hapalochlaenae*) and the rough-skinned newt (*Taricha granulosa*). It is not produced by the animals themselves but by symbiotic bacteria (certain species of *Pseudomonas* and *Vibrio*) that live within them. The toxin can be used either as a defensive or predatory venom and inhibits nerve activity by binding specifically in the external vestibule of the Na^+ channel and blocking ion permeation by occluding the channel pore. The pufferfish and other animals are not affected by the toxin because they carry a mutation in the protein sequence of their Na^+ channels that decreases the binding of the toxin. Its name is derived from *Tetraodontidae*; it was first isolated in 1894 and named in 1909 by Japanese scientist Yoshizumi Tahara. It is extremely toxic, roughly ten times more poisonous than potassium cyanide. Taken orally the LD_{50} for humans is about 25 mg but by injection about 0.6 mg. The dangers of eating pufferfish are noted in Egyptian hieroglyphs and described by Captain James Cook during his explorations of the South Seas in 1774. TTX is not affected by cooking and when inside the body does not cross the blood–brain barrier, but leaves the victim fully conscious while paralyzing the respiratory muscles. Death is due to asphyxia. Fugu is the Japanese word for pufferfish and the dish prepared from it is a delicacy in Japan. It must be carefully prepared to remove the toxic parts of the animal and to avoid these contaminating the rest of the fish. Most deaths from eating fugu occur when untrained people catch and prepare the fish. Poisoning does not always lead to death and sometimes imparts a numbness or tingling sensation on the lips and tongue which can be part of the appeal of eating this delicacy. Fugu is also the only food the Emperor of Japan is expressly forbidden to eat.

So the single-channel current produced by a driving force of 100 mV will be 10 pA. Recall also that one ampere is the flow of one coulomb of charge past a point in one second, so a current of 10 pA represents 10 pC of charge. One coulomb is equivalent to 6.2×10^{18} elementary charges (calculated by dividing Avogadro's number by the Faraday constant) so 62 million ions pass through a channel in 1 s.

4.7 Some channels can sense voltage

A sub-set of the channels have to be able to sense the voltage drop across the membrane in order for their function to be voltage dependent. In a moment we will look at the structure of some voltage-gated channels, showing how the main aspects of their function can be incorporated into a realistic and working picture. To enhance our understanding of how we arrived at these working models, we should briefly look at three different techniques that have been, and continue to be, used for elucidating channel structure/function relationships. The techniques fall into three broad categories:
(1) biophysical,
(2) molecular biological and
(3) microscopy, electron diffraction and cryo-electron microscopy.

4.8 Biophysical techniques – the patch clamp

It was not until a new technique called "patch clamp" was introduced in the 1970s and early 1980s that the properties of individual ionic channels ultimately responsible for the macroscopic currents could be worked out. Using this technique it is possible to record small currents that can be identified as flowing through single channels. The technique was developed by Erwin Neher and Bert Sakmann, and has proved so popular and has become so widely used that they received the Nobel Prize in 1991. Figure 4.1 illustrates the technique. A microelectrode connected via a $Ag^+/AgCl$ wire to an amplifier and a current–voltage convertor is pressed against a cell membrane and, with gentle suction, this forms a tight seal of very high resistance between the glass of the electrode and the cell membrane – a so-called "gigaohm seal" (Fig. 4.1B). The resistance associated with such a seal is at least 1 $G\Omega$, which is high enough to prevent significant current leaking across it so that current passing through the membrane patch containing a channel (or channels) is measured faithfully. Instead of voltage clamping the whole cell, a patch of membrane can be clamped, hence the term "patch clamp". If the channel of interest is in the patch of membrane then one can record its behaviour in response to voltage or other stimuli (Fig. 4.1C).

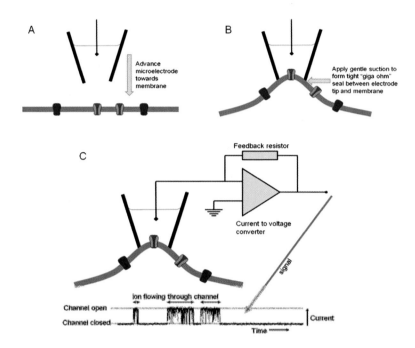

Figure 4.1. Panel A: A microelectrode filled with a suitable solution mimicking the intracellular environment is connected via a $Ag^+/AgCl$ wire to an amplifier and current–voltage convertor. Panel B: The microelectrode is pressed against a cell membrane and gentle suction applied to form a tight seal of very high resistance between the glass of the electrode and the cell membrane. The patch of membrane isolated by the electrode may contain one, a few or many channels. Panel C: Fluctuations in current take place as the channel opens and closes in response to voltage or other stimuli.

4.8.1 *Ensemble currents*

The cell-attached patch configuration isolates one or a few channels and allows recording of activity of those channels. The cell contents remain within the cell and the cytoplasm is not changed. The fluctuations in current take place as the channel opens and closes. The large macroscopic current measured by Hodgkin and Huxley is the result of many thousands of these microscopic currents flowing at the same time. For example, the behaviour of the macroscopic (or cellular) Na^+ current following a depolarizing pulse is the average of the individual responses

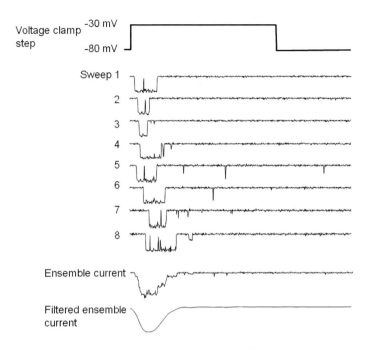

Figure 4.2. A series of eight patch electrode recordings of the response of a Na⁺ channel to a step change in voltage from –80 to –30 mV. Openings of the channels are observed as downward deflections in the traces. The mean or ensemble of the eight recording sweeps is shown and below that is the same trace having been filtered.

of the single channels to that depolarization. This behaviour can be seen in Fig. 4.2. The response in the lower part of Fig. 4.2 is the average current derived from the eight sweeps above it during the voltage changes illustrated at the top of the figure. This is known as an "ensemble current". Figure 4.2 illustrates that although individual channels open and close randomly, the probability that they are in the open state is greater when the membrane is more depolarized. The exact instant the channel will be open cannot be predicted. When the sweeps are averaged and one assumes the channels behave independently from each other, the response has a similar time course to the whole cell Na⁺ current, though it is much smaller. Notice that the single channels tend to open at the start of the depolarizing pulse and then they inactivate, entirely as predicted by Hodgkin and Huxley.

We can amend Eqn. 4.1 to take account of the concept that the macroscopic current, *I*, will reflect the current flowing through the single channel, *i*, times the number of channels in the membrane, *N*, times the probability that these are open, P_o:

$$I = i \times N_o \times P_o \qquad (4.3)$$

Ion channel gating typically tends to be modelled according to a "Markov process". This is a random process in which the state of a channel depends only on what is happening to it at the present time and not on events that took place prior to it arriving in its present state. In other words, the probability of a closed channel opening will be the same regardless of how long the channel was in the closed state. Ion channels do not have a "memory".

In Fig. 4.3A the single-channel currents are carried by K^+. When there is the same concentration of K^+ inside the pipette as outside and no potential across the membrane, no current flows. When +20 mV is applied to the pipette, this positive potential drives K^+ outwards. The channel randomly opens and closes and openings are observed as upward deflections on the traces. When –20 mV of voltage is applied to the pipette, K^+ is driven inward. The channel still randomly opens and closes but the openings are observed as downward deflections on the traces. As the applied potential is increased then the single-channel current becomes larger due to the large driving force. The relation between the size of the current and the voltage applied is linear and so the channel obeys Ohm's law. The slope of the relation graphed in Fig. 4.3B is determined by the concentration of the ions on either side of the channel and how quickly they pass through the channel. If the solutions on either side of the single channel contain more physiological values of $[K^+]$ (in this case, 140 mM K^+ on one side and 6 mM K^+ on the other), then the relation shifts to the left (Fig. 4.3B). The point at which the relation hits the *x*-axis, i.e. when the current moves from one that is inward to one that is outward, is the reversal potential (E_{rev}) – a term we already met in Chapter 2.

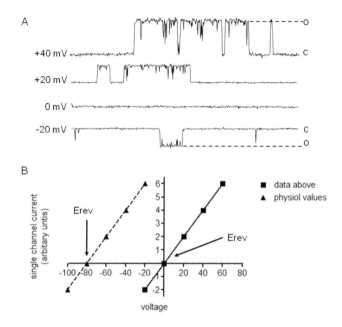

Figure 4.3. Panel A: Single-channel recordings of K^+ channel behaviour. The K^+ concentration is the same inside and outside the electrode. When there is no potential difference across the membrane, no current flows. When +20mV is applied to the pipette, K^+ is driven outwards when the channel randomly opens and closes. Openings are observed as upward deflections on the traces. When –20 mV of voltage is applied to the pipette, K^+ is driven inwards. The channel still randomly opens and closes but the openings are observed as downward deflections on the traces. When the potential difference is increased the single channel current becomes larger. Panel B shows the relation between the size of the current and the voltage applied. When the solutions bathing either side of the single-channel contain more physiological values of $[K^+]$ (140 mM and 6 mM), the relation shifts to the left. The points at which the relations intersect the x-axis are the reversal potentials, E_{rev}.

Since we know that:

$$V = I \times R \qquad (4.1)$$

and $1/R$ = conductance (G) then the slope of this relation is the channel conductance. If (say) the single-channel current averages 6 pA with 60 mV of potential applied across the membrane, then the conductance

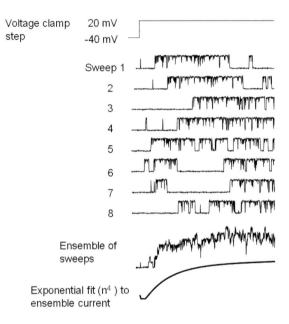

Figure 4.4. A series of eight patch electrode recordings of the response of a K^+ channel to a step change in voltage from –40 to +20 mV. Openings of the channels are observed as upward deflections in the traces. The mean or ensemble of the eight recording sweeps is shown and below that is a line of best fit (an exponential function).

is:

$$6 \ (pA)/60 \ (mV) = (6 \times 10^{-12})/(60 \times 10^{-3}) = 100 \ pS.$$

K^+ channels respond more slowly to depolarization than Na^+ channels and remain open for longer, as shown in Fig. 4.4. The average ensemble current shows similar characteristics to the delayed K^+ current observed by Hodgkin and Huxley.

4.8.2 *Other patch clamp configurations*

Various other patch clamp configurations can be used to allow access to the whole cell (Fig. 4.5A) or to the cytoplasmic face of the channels (Fig. 4.5B). A common form of patch clamp used in heart cell electrophysiology is the whole cell voltage clamp where a strong pulse of

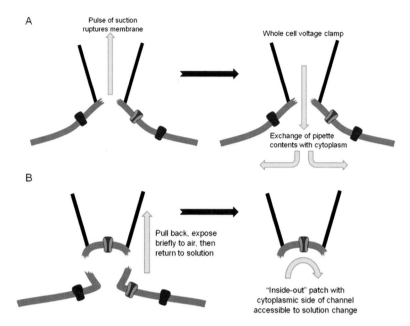

Figure 4.5. Other patch clamp configurations. Panel A: Rupturing the membrane with a pulse of suction allows access to the cell interior (so-called "whole cell" configuration) in which the contents of the electrode exchange with the cytoplasm of the cell. Panel B: Pulling the electrode back from the attached cell ruptures the membrane around the mouth of the electrode. Returning the electrode to the solution allows superfusion of the intracellular face of the channel protein.

suction is applied after forming a gigaohm seal. This ruptures the membrane and allows the whole cell to be voltage clamped. This allows macroscopic recording from all the channels in the cell and does not permit the activity of one or a few channels to be monitored. The cell contents are exchanged with the pipette solution and so the experimenter has a degree of control of the cytoplasmic solution. Patches of membrane containing one or a few channels can be pulled away from the cell and this provides access to their cytoplasmic face to assess the effects of a variety solutions and drugs that is not feasible in the other configurations.

4.9 Molecular techniques – working with frogs and fruit flies

4.9.1 *Frogs*

The oocytes of the African clawed frogs, *Xenopus laevis* and *Xenopus tropicalis,* are very large – about 1 mm in diameter – so they are easy to inject with heterologous cRNA, maintain in culture and voltage clamp (Fig. 4.6). They have become a widely used, controllable expression system for the characterization of ion channels. *Xenopus* oocytes translate cRNA very rapidly and effectively so a large number of copies of the ion channels thus encoded are generated and incorporated in their plasma membranes. Moreoever, the *Xenopus* oocytes do not have a large number of endogenous ion channels, and those that are expressed can be blocked at the translation stage by injection of antisense oligonucleotides into the oocyte so that currents arising from such channels – which could mask the function of the newly expressed ones – are greatly reduced. After a few hours or days, depending on the speed of expression of the channel, the follicular cell layers and connective tissue are removed by an enzyme treatment and the cell is voltage clamped by a two-electrode system. This allows the measurement of ion current flowing through the newly expressed channels.

Oocytes have been fundamental in examining the relationship between channel structure (i.e. its amino acid make-up) and function. This can be done very precisely, since sophisticated molecular biology techniques allow channel gene sequences to be changed deliberately so that the resulting expressed channel differs from the normal one by (say) one amino acid. The technique is called site-directed mutagenesis. Mutant forms of the channel can be expressed quickly in *Xenopus* oocytes and so the functional consequences of such mutations can be assessed to build a picture of how the channel's structure dictates the way it functions.

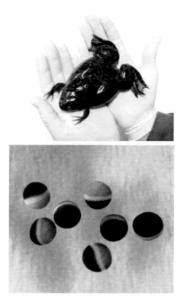

Figure 4.6. Upper panel: A *Xenopus* frog. Lower panel: *Xenopus* oocytes. With permission from Xenopus Express Inc. and Drs Silke Haerteis and Matteus Krappitz, University of Erlangen-Nürnberg.

4.9.2 *Fruit flies*

The first channel gene cloned was one that codes for a particular family of voltage-dependent potassium ion channels in the fruit fly, *Drosophila melanogaster* (see Fig. 4.7). Mutations of this gene caused alterations to the fly's behaviour especially under ether anaesthesia. Predominant amongst a variety of strange movements was the shaking of the fly's legs. The gene was therefore called the Shaker (Sh) gene. The flies with the mutant gene have a shorter lifespan than normal flies and their larvae show repetitive firing of action potentials in neurons and at neuromuscular junctions. The cloning of the Sh gene and development of Sh mutants allowed us to examine how ion channel structure and function influences behaviour, neural and synaptic physiology.

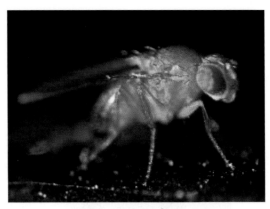

Figure 4.7. *Drosophila melanogaster.*

The Shaker channel of *Drosophila* turned out to be the archetypal K$^+$ channel. Its cloning led to the identification of members of a superfamily of homologous K$^+$ channels in vertebrates, namely the voltage sensitive, or K$_V$, channels. The Shaker gene encodes the α-subunit of the channel that consists of the six transmembrane-spanning segments which we will consider elsewhere.

A working Shaker channel has four subunits that form the pore and carries A-type K$^+$ current responsible for repolarizing the cell. Certain mutations in the Sh gene reduce the conductance of this channel type in the neuronal membrane impairing nerve repolarization, impulse propagation and synaptic function. These functional changes cause the severe phenotypical behaviour and movement patterns.

The Sh gene is located on the X-chromosome and encodes a large transcriptional unit (>110 kb of DNA). Alternative splicing of the RNA can generate many RNA transcripts coding for protein isoforms, which may have different functional characteristics and be expressed in different amounts depending on the tissue (Fig. 4.8). The transcripts tend to have a conserved main region (grey bar) and variable 5′ (amino) and 3′ (carboxy) ends.

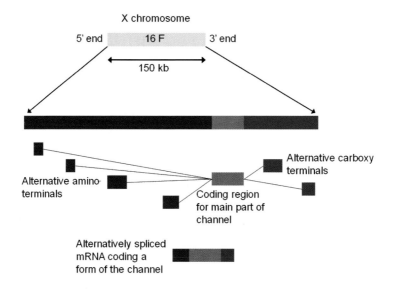

Figure 4.8. An illustration of how alternative splicing of precursor RNA can generate many RNA transcripts coding for channel isoforms which may have different functional characteristics. The corresponding protein isoforms translated from the mRNA shown here will have different N- and C-terminals.

Alternative splicing of precursor RNA enables a single gene to encode multiple protein isoforms with different functional characteristics and tissue distributions.

4.10 Microscopy, electron diffraction and cryo-electron microscopy

Like many molecules, proteins can form crystals given the right conditions. To crystallize a protein, the purified protein must be slowly precipitated from an aqueous solution so that the molecules align in a repeating series with consistent orientation – the so-called crystal "lattice". If crystals are produced without contaminants and large enough to provide an X-ray diffraction pattern, then the pattern can be analysed to determine the protein's three-dimensional structure. Protein crystallization is inherently difficult because peptides tend to be flexible and do not have a preferable conformation, and their crystals are fragile compared with those of inorganic salts. Successfully creating protein crystals that are suitable for X-ray diffraction analyses is dependent on luck, experience and a number of environmental factors.

Commonly used methods for protein crystallization are variations of vapour diffusion. A droplet containing purified protein, buffer and precipitant is allowed to equilibrate with a larger reservoir containing the same buffer and precipitant but in greater concentration. As water vaporizes from the drop and transfers to the reservoir, the precipitant concentration increases to a point where crystals start to form. These crystals need to be large enough to diffract X-rays and form a detectable pattern, but small enough not to become distorted. The optimal size is about 0.1–1.0 mm. The crystals are mounted on a support and placed on the detector under the X-ray beam with fine attention paid to the geometry of the experiment. The X-ray data are then processed and scaled and the emerging protein structure refined.

Another technique used to probe channel protein structure is cryo-electron microscopy or cryo-EM. Samples of the protein are frozen in an ethane slush to produce vitreous, or non-crystalline, ice. The frozen sample is then analysed at very low temperature (liquid nitrogen) in the electron microscope. The main advantage of cryo-EM over traditional EM techniques is that the sample is preserved in its native hydrated state without it being distorted by stains or fixatives usually associated with traditional EM. The sample is always in solution so its shape is maintained and also not distorted by attachment to a support structure. With image processing and averaging a great many images, cryo-EM provides high-resolution information (below 10 Å).

4.11   More understanding of channel structure and function

By using all these techniques we are beginning to understand the structure of some channels and appreciate how they function. We now recognize that there is wide channel diversity even within groups of channels that conduct the same ion, K^+ channels for example. Channel proteins also vary greatly in size. At one extreme, Gramicidin D, an antibiotic compound, is 15 amino acids long and dimerizes to form a channel, while the sarcoplasmic Ca^{2+} release channel (also known as the ryanodine receptor) is around 5000 amino acids long and has many subunits and regulatory sites.

By 1980 we also knew that at least some ion channels consisted of more than a single protein subunit. One of the first descriptions of a multimeric channel protein complex was produced for the nicotinic acetylcholine receptor. The receptor is essentially a ligand-gated ion channel consisting of five subunits (α, β, γ, δ and ε) arranged around a central pore region. In the neuronal form of the receptor, the acetylcholine binding site is formed by groups of amino acid residues from the α and β subunits. When an agonist (normally acetylcholine) binds to the site, all the subunits undergo conformational changes and the central channel opens. (This channel is unlike many others we will describe later in that it is permeable to both Na^+ and K^+. However, when the post-synaptic cell is polarized normally at its resting membrane potential, the binding of ACh produces a depolarization mainly due to Na^+ influx).

4.12 Channel subunits

Subunits of channels seem to be important in modulating their function and allowing them to signal and interact with other proteins in the cell. The main subunit that forms the channel pore is often called the α-subunit. It may be capable of forming a functioning channel on its own but may need other subunits to combine to form a fully working channel. Other subunits forming what is usually a heteromeric channel complex are generally referred to by the Greek letters β, γ, δ etc. An example of a channel in the heart that requires subunit interaction to form a fully functioning structure is one that carries potassium current (called I_{Ks}) and activates slowly. Channels that give rise to I_{Ks} are formed by an α-subunit called KCNQ1 (the description of the gene that codes for the subunit) which is 676 amino acids long and a smaller peptide of 129 amino acids that has one trans-membrane domain called MinK (also known as KCNE1, again, the description of the gene that codes for the smaller peptide). The MinK subunit confers subtle functions to the α-complex by influencing gating kinetics, unitary conductance and the binding of drugs. Channels formed from KCNQ1 alone activate rapidly, exhibit current saturation and have a small single-channel conductance. In contrast, when the channels are formed with MinK they activate more slowly, do not saturate with prolonged depolarization, have a larger unitary conductance, have better ion discrimination and are responsive to a variety of activators and inhibitors.

4.13   Channel structure

4.13.1   *Protein structure – a recap*

The primary structure of the proteins determines their secondary structure since certain amino acids combine to form stable α-helices (e.g. alanine and leucine) whilst others form unstable bonds (e.g. serine and isoleucine). From the primary sequence it is possible to predict regions of the protein molecule that are likely to form α-helices or β-pleated sheets (see Fig. 4.9). It is also possible to predict how hydrophobic these secondary structures are. Depending on the charge on the side chain of the component amino acids, polypeptide secondary structure can have hydrophobic or hydrophilic properties. These are important in forming the tertiary protein structure (and also in quaternary protein–protein interactions). Clusters of hydrophobic amino acids grouped together often indicate a portion of the polypeptide that traverses the lipid membrane.

In an α-helix that spans the membrane, the intra-membrane segment will have amino acid side groups that protrude from the helically coiled polypeptide backbone which are largely hydrophobic, so that interactions with membrane lipids are maximized resulting in a more stable molecule. The polar parts of the peptide molecule remain buried within the helical backbone. Amino acids with aliphatic (no ring compounds – benzene etc.) side chains (leucine, isoleucine, alanine, valine) are hydrophobic and there is a preponderance of these in the middle of the bilayer.

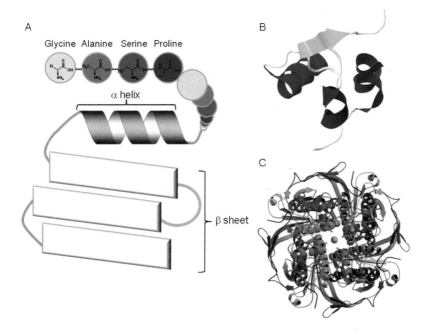

Figure 4.9. The building blocks of protein structure. Panel A: The primary structure is the amino acid sequence of the peptide chain which can form regular structures using hydrogen bonding called α-helices and β-sheets. Panel B: α-helices and β-sheets can fold into complex, three-dimensional tertiary structures using a variety of bonding. Panel C: The three-dimensional tertiary structures group to form a multi-subunit protein with quaternary structure.

On the other hand, lysine and arginine are often at the lipid/water interface, where the positively charged groups at the ends of their aliphatic side chains make stable interactions with the polar membrane components at the surface. It is possible to make assessments of the relative hydrophobicity of sequences of amino acid residues in the form of hydropathy plots to help predict the probability of an α-helix or β-sheet forming a trans-membrane domain. The plots are also referred to as Kyte–Doolittle plots after the two people who popularized their use. Hydropathy analyses search for clusters of 20 or so linked amino acids with predominantly hydrophobic residues. This is because α-helices of 20 amino acids in length are just long enough to span a lipid bilayer. Many putative hydrophobic trans-membrane α-helices have been

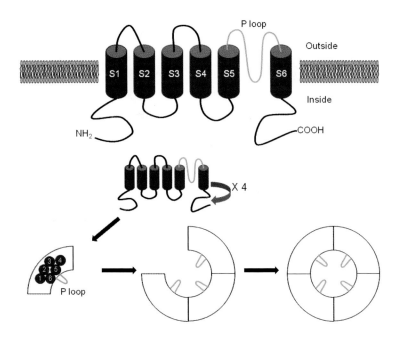

Figure 4.10. The structure typical of a voltage-gated K^+ channel. The channel comprises four α-subunit proteins each consisting of six membrane-spanning α-helical segments, S1 to S6. The amino- or N-terminal and carboxy- or C-terminal of the subunits are intracellular. The channel is formed by the association of identical subunits (homomeric) or by different ones (heteromeric). Part of the protein between S5 and S6 does not fully traverse the membrane and is called the P loop. It forms a specialized part of the channel involved in ion conduction and selection.

identified this way. It is then possible to begin to make a few basic predictions of how the secondary structures might fold to form three-dimensional tertiary ones and, along with more complex protein-folding algorithms run on a computer, forecast channel structures.

4.13.2 *K^+ channel structure*

The first channel structure we will show in detail in Fig. 4.10 is typical of voltage-gated K^+ channels. The structure is an assembly of four α-subunit proteins each consisting of six membrane-spanning α-helical segments, S1 to S6. The beginning (amino- or N-terminal) and end

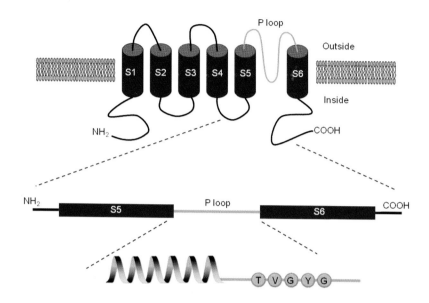

Figure 4.11. The conserved sequence of five amino acids in the P loop. T, threonine; V, valine; G, glycine and Y, tyrosine.

(carboxy- or C-terminal) of the subunits are intracellular. The channel pore is formed by the association of identical subunits (homomeric) or by different ones (heteromeric) with its narrowest part, termed the selectivity filter, being formed by a loop that dips into the membrane but does not fully cross it between the trans-membrane helices S5 and S6. The short loop is called the "P loop" (sometimes referred to as "2TM/P") and appears to be a universal feature of K^+ channels as there is a conserved sequence of five amino acids, threonine (Thr), valine (Val), glycine (Gly), tyrosine (Tyr) and another Gly in many channels (i.e. similar or identical sequences) (Fig. 4.11). This TVGYG sequence, as we will see, allows the channels to discriminate between different ions. Functionally, this type of channel produces the voltage- and Ca^{2+}-activated groups of K^+ channels but there are many variations of this basic K^+ channel architecture. Channels can also be formed from a tetrameric clustering of subunits with two membrane-spanning segments.

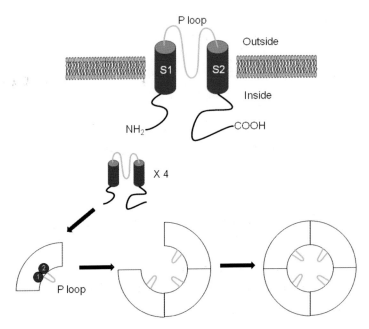

Figure 4.12. The structure typical of inward-rectifying K^+ channels. The channel comprises four α-subunit proteins each consisting of two membrane-spanning α-helical segments, S1 and S2.

These have a P loop and gross structure analogous to the S5–P–S6 grouping of the S1–S6 channel subunits. Such assemblies produce the inward-rectifying K channels (Fig. 4.12). A third group of subunits contain four membrane-spanning segments (M1–M4) and have two P loops (P1 and P2). It is thought that only two subunits form a functional channel or, if four subunits co-assemble, then a complex with two pores forms. Currents flowing through these channels are not voltage dependent, are not inhibited by conventional K^+ channel blockers and are often described as "background" or "leak" K^+ channels.

In three dimensions the voltage-dependent K^+ channels formed by the assembly of the six membrane-spanning α-helical segments, S1 to S6, look like those shown in Fig. 4.13. These K^+ channels were produced in COS cells, purified on an immunoaffinity column and studied with an

(a)

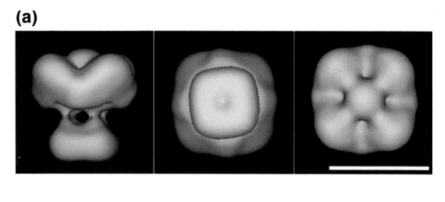

(b)

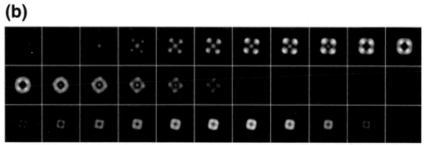

Figure 4.13. A surface representation of the three-dimensional structure of the Shaker channel elucidated using cryo-EM. Panel A shows three views of the channel in different orientations. Left: The channel axis is in the plane of the image with the membrane domain up and the cytoplasmic domain down, Middle: Facing the cytoplasmic domain (i.e. from the bottom), Right: Facing the membrane domain (i.e. from the top). Scale bar is 10 nm. Panel B shows slices (each 0.35 nm) through the channel perpendicular to its axis of symmetry. Slices start at the top left from the membrane domain. Reproduced from Sokolova *et al.* (2001). *Structure* **9**, 215–220 with permission.

electron microscope. The structure has a square shape and clearly shows two domains linked by thin connectors about 2 nm long. The larger domain (normally embedded in the membrane) is about 10 nm across and 6 nm thick and the smaller domain (normally free in the cytoplasm) is about 6 nm across and 3 nm thick. The larger domain probably represents the main channel and the smaller one is involved with regulation and inactivation of the channel.

So we now know that channels can:

(1) be voltage gated
(2) have high transport rates or throughput
(3) discriminate between certain ions and
(4) function independently carrying specific ionic species

We will now examine the structural basis for these features.

4.14   The structural basis of ion channel function

4.14.1   *Sensing the voltage across the cell membrane*

(1) A sub-set of the channels have to be able to sense the voltage drop across the membrane in order for their function to be voltage dependent.

The fourth trans-membrane segment (S4) span of each monomer of the K^+ channel has highly conserved sequences of amino acids with 5–7 arginine residues that are positively charged at physiological pH. Sometimes the arginine is replaced by lysine, but there appear to be about five to seven elementary charges on each S4 segment. Mutations in this domain (often by only a single amino acid) cause changes in the voltage dependence of the channel.

It is thought that S4 with part of S3 forms a so-called "voltage-sensor paddle" on the outside of the channel protein at the interface between it and the lipid bilayer on the cytoplasmic surface and moves akin to a ratchet mechanism in response to the changes in electric field across the membrane (Fig. 4.14). As the membrane depolarizes, the four paddles (one on each monomer) move through the membrane tugging on the linking element between S4 and S5 (aptly named the "S4–S5 linker"). This, in turn, pulls the S5 helices away from the pore which, along with induced movement of S6, opens the channel (Fig. 4.15 and Fig. 4.16). The voltage-sensor paddles move in atomic terms quite a large distance – about 20 Å – nearly perpendicular to the membrane surface. The gates to the channel vestibule are the S6 helices and these splay open to allow

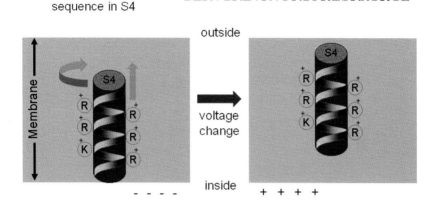

Conserved amino acid sequence in S4

ILRVIRLVRVFRIFKLSRHSKGL

Figure 4.14. How the domain with a highly conserved sequence of arginine residues may respond to a voltage change across the cell membrane. R, arginine.

ions access to the vestibule. To splay apart, the S6 helices need to bend and in bacterial K^+ channels a highly conserved glycine residue appears to provide the necessary hinge point (the so-called glycine hinge). If this glycine residue is point mutated the channels lock in a closed state. In eukaryotic K^+ channels, S6 hinges at a proline–valine–proline sequence. In this way the channel "gates" open and provide access for the ions in solution to the inner selectivity pore (Fig. 4.15 and Fig. 4.16). There are other models of voltage sensing that differ slightly in the way and amount that S4 moves. The paddle model description used here illustrates the concepts involved – it may not be an exact description of how all channels gate.

4.14.2 *Moving ions into the channel*

(2) Channels have high throughput.

Having the channel open allows ions to move through it, so providing a pathway for the selected ion (in this case K^+) to progress according to its electrochemical gradient across the dielectric barrier of the phospholipid membrane. How does the ion overcome the dielectric barrier?

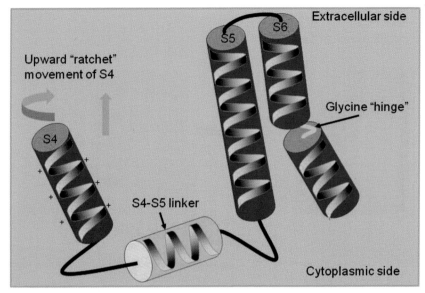

Figure 4.15. Movement of S4. As S4 moves through the membrane it tugs on the linking element between S4 and S5. This pulls the S5 helices away from the pore and induces movement of S6, which probably bends at the glycine hinge to open the channel.

The movement of residues as the channel opens creates a large (at least 12 Å wide) cytoplasmic cavity surrounded by four α-helices associated with the P loop, termed "pore helices", which have their carboxy terminals positioned towards the centre of the water-filled cavity. The negative charges on these carboxyl groups stabilize an ion whilst it is residing in the cavity (Fig. 4.17). Since it is (again atomically speaking) quite wide, the cavity becomes continuous with the intracellular solution and so greatly lowers the access resistance for a K^+ ion diffusing between the cytoplasm and the inner part of the conduction pathway or "selectivity filter". This increases the probability of an ion moving from the cytoplasm to the cavity and enlarges the channels' so-called "capture radius". Further, in the open conformation, the channel effectively thins the membrane for a diffusing ion to pass through, essentially to the length of the inner conduction pathway, a characteristic that allows ions to diffuse very rapidly across about half the membrane bilayer before reaching the selectivity filter. Together, these features

Closed channel

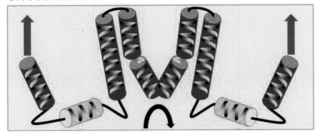

K⁺ entry to channel impeded

Open channel

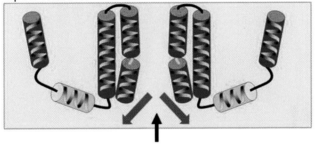

K⁺ can enter channel

Figure 4.16. S4 moves upwards through the membrane tugging the linking element and S5. This induces movement of S6 which hinges and the channel opens to provide access for the ions in solution to the inner selectivity pore.

assist K^+ channels in grabbing, stabilizing and initiating the transfer of ions, which partly contributes to them having very high conductances.

The wide diameter of the cavity also explains Hagiwara and Armstrong's much earlier observations with quaternary ammonium compounds. On its cytoplasmic side the open channel is wide enough to allow these compounds to lodge in the cavity and stop conduction of the ion through the selectivity filter. This also may explain why many K^+ channels are susceptible to blocking by a variety of prescription medicines that give rise to drug-induced cardiac arrhythmias and conduction abnormalities. These drugs tend to block the channel by occupying the cavity.

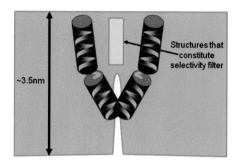

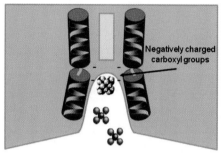

Figure 4.17.   An indication of how the cytoplasmic cavity forms as the channel opens is achieved by showing a slice through the K channel. The blue shading corresponds to the channel protein with the positions of S6 superimposed. The white regions in the figure correspond to aqueous solution. The channel protein is roughly 35 Å (3.5 nm) in its trans-membrane dimension.   Two pore helices are shown, the other two are in front and behind the plane of the illustration. A tetraethylammonium (TEA^+) ion (grey) is shown in the cavity blocking the progress of two hydrated K^+ ions upwards towards the selectivity filter.

4.14.3 *Discriminating between ions*

(3) Ion channels are discerning.

We calculated earlier in the chapter that about 62 million K^+ ions can pass through a channel in 1 s. Knowing this allows us to pose the obvious question: how are K^+ channels able to achieve this fast throughput of ions whilst being at least 1000 times more selective for K^+ over Na^+? The selectivity and throughput processes are even more demanding because the atomic radius of K^+ is 1.33 Å whereas that of Na^+

is 0.95 Å. In other words, K^+ is the larger atom yet the channel transports it rapidly but blocks the smaller one. The way the channel selects ions is based on differences in the free energy of hydration between K^+ and Na^+ – an idea that was gradually modified by Eisenman and Bezanilla and Armstrong over several years from the early 1970s.

To understand what is happening we need to know a little about how ions dissolve in water. When a salt is dissolved in water it dissociates into its component anions and cations. Water molecules are very strongly attracted to the ions forming a primary solvation shell around them. In this shell the oxygen atoms of the water molecules donate both their electrons to form a covalent bond with the ion. The strength of the ion–oxygen bond is generally greater when the charge on the ion is greater and less as the size of the ion increases, but in most cases is very strong giving a stable electrostatic ion–water interaction. The water molecules bonded to the ion can also be attached by hydrogen bonds to other water molecules just outside the solvation shell, so that in dilute solutions the shell merges into the water structure.

The solvation shells are in a constant state of change whereby water molecules binding to the ions are frequently being substituted (on a nanosecond timescale) by other neighbouring molecules. This constant movement arises from thermal agitation and is an important aspect to grasp as we explore the movement of ions through the selectivity filter of a channel.

Working out the three-dimensional structure of a K^+ channel was a huge step forward in understanding how ions move through it. This major tour-de-force was achieved by Rod MacKinnon and colleagues, who produced crystals of a bacterial K^+ channel called "KcsA", which they then studied at a very high resolution of 3 Å. For this work MacKinnon was awarded the Nobel Prize in 2003. This channel molecule became their primary focus because the large quantity of channel protein needed for crystallography could be obtained by growing large numbers of bacteria (*Streptomyces lividans*) expressing this molecule. The KcsA channel has a simpler structure compared with other K^+ channels in that it has only two membrane-spanning segments per

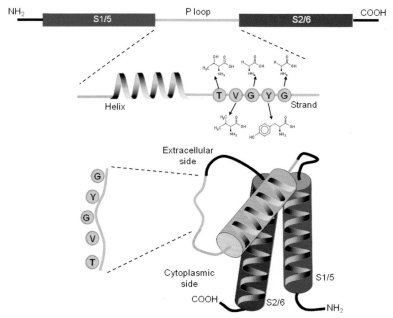

Figure 4.18. The signature sequence in the P loop. T, threonine; V, valine; G, glycine and Y, tyrosine.

subunit, which correspond to the S5, P loop and S6 areas of the larger six trans-membrane domain subunit structure and are designated S1/5 and S2/6 in Fig. 4.18. Despite it being of bacterial origin, KcsA closely resembles the amino acid sequence of the pore of the larger eukaryotic K^+ channel proteins and shares similar pharmacological properties. Armed with the knowledge that mutations of certain amino acids within the P loop affected the channel's ability to discriminate between K^+ and Na^+ ions and the burgeoning amount of molecular biology studies of K^+ channels showing a strikingly common sequence of amino acids within the loop, MacKinnon deduced that this highly conserved segment of the protein was important for K^+ channel selectivity. He called these amino acids the "signature sequence of the K^+ channel" and imagined the tetrameric formation of the four pore loops in some way produce a pore with the signature sequence of amino acids lining it (Fig. 4.18). He then showed, in a groundbreaking series of papers between 1998 and 2001,

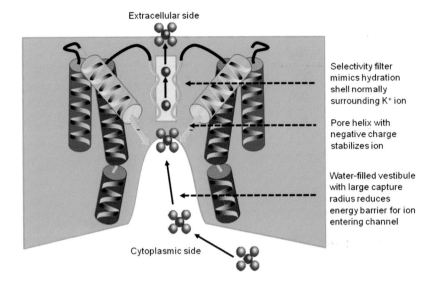

Extracellular side

Selectivity filter mimics hydration shell normally surrounding K⁺ ion

Pore helix with negative charge stabilizes ion

Water-filled vestibule with large capture radius reduces energy barrier for ion entering channel

Cytoplasmic side

Figure 4.19. A hydrated K^+ ion is "captured" by the water-filled vestibule which reduces the energy barrier for an ion approaching the channel. As the ion leaves the inner vestibule and enters the selectivity filter the pore helices stabilize it. The solvation shell normally surrounding the ion is then replaced by oxygen atoms from the selectivity portion of the channel, which make an ideal chemical and energetic match.

that the three-dimensional structure of the KcsA protein contained such a pore, which lay along the axis of symmetry of the tetramer at the shared interface of the four subunits and had all the necessary architecture required to stabilize and assist the passage of a K^+ ion through the channel.

The pore area contains four K^+ binding sites in a row (numbered 4, 3, 2, 1 from inside the cell to outside), forming the selectivity filter. At each of these sites, a K^+ ion is dehydrated and interacts with eight charged oxygen atoms that coordinate with the K^+ ions (see Fig. 4.20). When the ion leaves the inner vestibule and enters the selectivity filter, the solvation shell normally surrounding the K^+ ion is replaced by oxygen atoms from the protein, which make an ideal chemical and energetic match (Fig. 4.19). As MacKinnon states, this structure keeps the K^+ ion

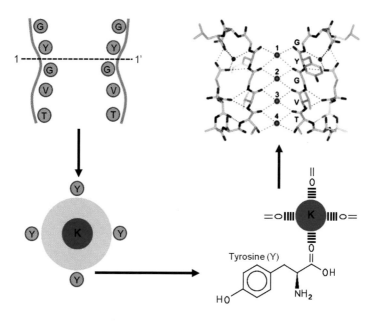

Figure 4.20. Coordination of the K^+ ion through the selectivity filter. Top left: the highly conserved segment of the protein important for K^+ channel selectivity is formed by the TVGYG sequence. The filter pore is formed from four loops, two of which are shown here. Bottom left and right: slicing (1 – 1′) through the pore and looking from above, the K^+ ion coordinates with the oxygen groups lining the pore. Top right: eight oxygen groups coordinate with each ion at four binding sites numbered 4–1 from inside the cell to outside.

"comfortable" by taking the place of its hydration shell while it moves through the selectivity filter. For an ion to enter the pore, it must shed the water molecules forming its solvation shell because only non-hydrated K^+ ions can fit in.

Larger cations, such as Cs^+, cannot fit through the pore, though smaller ones, such as Na^+, can. However, nature has designed the system very cleverly because, although Na^+ ions can pass through the filter, their passage is much more energetically unfavourable because the binding sites are too far apart to perfectly stabilize a dehydrated Na^+ ion (Figs.

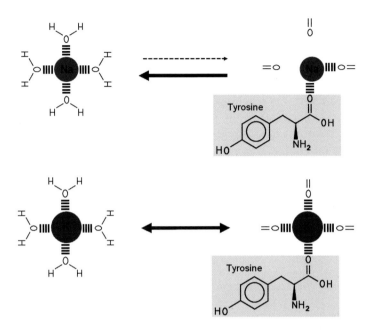

Figure 4.21. In the lower panel the K^+ ion is fully hydrated by six (only four are drawn here) water molecules (left). On the right is shown what happens at each of the binding sites in the selectivity pore. The K^+ ion is dehydrated and interacts with eight charged oxygen atoms (four from each site above and below it). The oxygen atoms coordinate with the K^+ ion akin to the water molecules, providing the ideal chemical and energetic match so binding is in equilibrium. The oxygen atoms are provided by the key amino acids that line the selectivity pore (here for example is tyrosine). In the upper panel a Na^+ ion is also hydrated in the same way (left). It is small enough to be able to pass through the pore but the binding sites are too far apart to fully stabilize the dehydrated ion, so passage through the pore is much more energetically unfavourable.

4.20 and 4.21). In other words, Na^+ ions are too small to fit effortlessly in the coordination cage provided by the channel pore and so the energy demands of dehydrating these smaller ions are just too great and result in their exclusion. The selectivity filter is about 12 Å in length and is the channel's discrimination mechanism. It is about the same length as the inner water-filled vestibule which forms when the channel opens and together, these architectural elements allow high ion flux rates.

When the channel is open at physiological K^+ concentrations the pore is usually occupied by two K^+ ions, (either at sites 1 and 3 or at 2 and 4 – Fig. 4.21). Dictated by mass action, a third ion will hop from the inner vestibule onto site 4 and the two ions already in the selectivity filter will be forced to move along the sites analogously to hopping over stepping stones in a river. On reaching the end of the line of binding sites the ion will rapidly dissociate from the channel complex and take up a new solvation shell. This Newton's cradle-like knock-on mechanism (in part conceived by Hodgkin and Keynes in 1955), whereby the binding of an incoming K^+ ion results in the ejection of another ion at the extracellular side of the pore, is the process that leads to the conduction of a single K^+ ion from one side of the membrane to the other.

4.15 Na^+ channels

(4) Channels function independently carrying specific ionic species.

Over the next few years, the depiction of KcsA structure was followed by even higher resolution images of it and other K^+ channels, allowing better predictions about the conduction and gating of this channel family. The work from the MacKinnon lab showed us what ion channels look like and from that we can begin to understand how they function. Structural and experimental evidence suggests that the KcsA channel is an evolutionary predecessor of the six trans-membrane segment family of voltage-gated K^+ channels. It is likely that voltage-gated Na^+ channels have evolved from K^+ channels by gene duplication, so whilst the pores and filters of the Na^+ channels must be structurally different, similar features governing permeation and selectivity in K^+ channels are likely to be present.

In 1984, Numa's laboratory in Kyoto were first to deduce the primary structure of the Na^+ channel isolated from the eel (*Electrophorus electricus*) and this was followed by publication of a variety of isoforms of the channel α-subunit which is roughly 2 000 amino acids long. The primary sequence of the human cardiac isoform was reported in 1992. Given its very specific action, TTX binding to the outer part of the

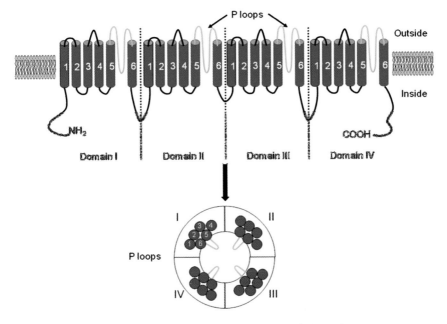

Figure 4.22. The α-subunit of a typical Na$^+$ channel.

channel was examined and modelled extensively because its interactions with this part of the channel allowed predictions to be made about the channel architecture needed to bind the structure.

The first reports of the crystal structure of a voltage-gated Na$^+$ channel from another type of bacteria, *Arcobacter butzleri* (NavAb), have been published quite recently. The Catterall group have made a thorough analysis of the three-dimensional structure of NavAb at 2.7 Å resolution, allowing a much better understanding of the structural features that are important for voltage-dependent gating, ion selectivity and drug block in Na$^+$ and also Ca^{2+} channels. The α-subunit of a typical Na$^+$ channel is about four times larger than the individual subunit of the K$^+$ channel and is depicted in Fig. 4.22. It has four homologous domains, each containing six membrane-spanning regions, so it resembles an amalgamation of the four subunits of the typical K$^+$

channel. Therefore, Na^+ channels are formed by one of these proteins whereas K^+ channels form by a grouping of four individual proteins.

The Na^+ channel pore-forming domain has similarities to the KcsA channel pore in that it is formed by a folding of S5, the P loop and S6 that correspond with the two trans-membrane and P domains of the latter. The outer vestibule is thought to be wider than that of KcsA in order to accommodate the large TTX molecule. The side chains of certain amino acid residues, instead of the main chain carbonyls in KcsA, form the selectivity filter. Point mutations in the Na^+ channel P loop show that key residues affect the conductance of the channel, its selectivity and its interaction with TTX. These experiments and close attention to amino acid alignment pointed to a cluster of four highly conserved amino acids in the same relative positions in the P loops of the four domains I–IV. Akin to the conserved primary sequence of TVGYG characterizing K^+ channels, Na^+ channels also appear to have a "signature pattern" comprising key amino acids believed to form the selectivity filter. They are aspartic acid (Asp or D) at amino acid (aa) 400, glutamic acid (Glu or E) at aa755, lysine (Lys or K) at aa1237 and alanine (Ala or A) at aa1529, and together they give rise to the term, DEKA motif. Na^+ channels are more selective for Na^+ (and other small ions such as Li^+) than larger monovalent cations (such as K^+, Cs^+ and Rb^+). Fozzard and colleagues propose that the Na^+ channel selectivity arises from electrostatic competition between the ion and the glutamic acid (in domain II) and lysine (in domain III) residues in the DEKA motif. Larger cations (such as K^+ and Rb^+) do not compete as successfully and this inhibits their permeation. Selectivity is not determined so much by the size of the pore at this point, more by the ability of the permeating ion to compete with the amino group on the lysine.

4.16 Channel inactivation

The structural studies help us to understand another gating process, namely, inactivation. K^+ channels that carry A-type current (such as the Shaker K^+ channel) and Na^+ and Ca^{2+} channels open in response to membrane depolarization but some milliseconds later they stop conducting ions. Recall that Hodgkin and Huxley described this process in terms of an *h* parameter that reacted to a voltage change more slowly than the initial opening of the channel. They envisaged the processes of activation and inactivation involving the sequential movement of particles.

Around 1977, Armstrong and colleagues proposed an explanation of Na^+ channel inactivation called the "ball and chain" mechanism. The idea was that, following the channel opening, a "ball" of channel peptide tethered to a "chain" of longer peptide that in turn was attached to the main pore-forming subunits swung into the channel from the cytoplasmic side and blocked ion movement through the pore. It was found that Na^+ channel inactivation could be removed by applying proteolytic enzymes to the intracellular surface yet the activation mechanism remained intact. This strongly suggested that activation and inactivation were separate mechanisms. Another line of evidence came from Armstrong's experiments on K^+ channels using derivatives of TEA with long side chains of seven or more methyl groups forming an ion with a charged head and a hydrophobic tail. The compounds blocked K^+ channels but only after the channels had been activated, so the blocking event was very similar to normal inactivation. Together, these types of experiment showed that a piece of the channel protein crucial for inactivation could be selectively removed without affecting the opening process and the action of these portions of protein could be mimicked by larger charged molecules. Adding to the picture, Lenaeus and colleagues showed that TEA blocks from the cytoplasmic side of the channel at the entrance to the selectivity filter and is stabilized by the hydrophobic residues of the inner helices. Once TEA is present in the channel it then cannot inactivate, suggesting the inactivation process needs access to the area near the inner helices.

The molecular details of this "ball and chain" inactivation mechanism were characterized by Aldrich working with colleagues Hoshi and Zagotta in the late 1980s and early 1990s. They studied the rapidly inactivating Shaker K^+ channel and showed that mutations of the channel (either deletions or substitutions of the first 19 amino acids at the NH_2

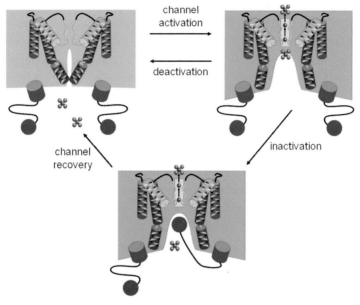

Figure 4.23. The inactivation process of a K^+ channel.

terminal of the protein) disrupted the inactivation process. In another experiment they expressed (in *Xenopus* oocytes) mutant channels that did not inactivate. They then made a synthetic peptide comprising the first 20 amino acids of the NH_2 terminal of normal Shaker K^+ channels and applied this intracellularly to the oocytes. The presence of the peptide restored inactivation in a concentration-dependent manner. These experiments provided very strong evidence that when a K^+ channel that shows inactivation is open, a peptide ball (made up of about 19 amino acids) tethered to the channel by a chain (made up of about 60 amino acids) formed either by the channel's own amino or N-terminal or an associated β-subunit moves into the mouth of the channel and blocks it, as depicted in Fig. 4.23. The inactivation of Na^+ channels takes place using an analogous process but involves a "hinged lid" rather than a ball and chain. The hinged lid is made from a loop of peptide linking the S3 and S4 domains and controls the exit of Na^+ from the channel into the cell.

4.17 Other ways of altering channel function

Finally in this chapter we should note that experiments by Levitan and others produced compelling evidence that phosphorylation (and dephosphorylation) of channel proteins affect their function. A diverse array of kinase signalling pathways phosphorylate ion channels resulting in some being activated and others being inhibited. This "post-translational processing" provides another route whereby channel function can be modulated.

4.18 Questions

(1) How would you determine the number of active channels of a particular type in a particular ventricular myocyte when it is clamped at a certain voltage? (Hint: think about macroscopic and microscopic currents.)

(2) Using patch recording, you determine the conductance (γ) for a specific Na^+ channel to be 30 pS (3.0×10^{-11} siemens). If the peak of the Na^+ current in the whole cell at –15 mV is 2 nA (2.0×10^{-9} A), what is the total number of Na^+ channels in the whole cell?

(3) A channel is open ten times per second. Each opening lasts an average of 20 ms. What is the open probability of this channel?

(4) A channel is selective for a monovalent cation with an equilibrium potential of –100 mV. The conductance of the channel is 100 pS. How many charges pass through the channel during a 200 ms clamp step when the membrane potential is held at –70 mV?

(5) If a channel is ligand gated, what are the factors that determine whether or not it is open?

4.19 Bibliography

4.19.1 *Books and reviews*

Bezanilla, F. (2000). The voltage sensor in voltage-dependent ion channels. *Physiol. Rev.* **80**, 556–592.

Gulbis, J.M. and Doyle, D.A. (2004). Potassium channel structures: do they conform? *Curr. Opin. Struct. Biol.* **14**, 440–446.

Hille, B., Armstrong, C.M. and MacKinnon, R. (1999). Ion channels: from idea to reality. *Nature Medicine* **5**, 1105–1109.

Hille, B. (2001). *Ion Channels of Excitable Membranes* 3rd edn. Sinauer Associates Inc.

Levitan, I.B. (1994). Modulation of ion channels by protein phosphorylation and dephosphorylation. *Ann. Rev. Physiol.* **56**, 193–212.

MacKinnon, R. (2003) [Online] Nobel Lecture. Available at: http://nobelprize.org/chemistry/laureates/2003/mackinnon-lecture.html.

Miller, C. (2000). Ion channels: doing hard chemistry with hard ions. *Curr. Opin. Chem. Biol.* **4**, 148–151.

Sakmann, B. and Neher, E. (1984). Patch clamp techniques for studying ionic channels in excitable membranes. *Ann. Rev. Physiol.* **46**, 455–472.

4.19.2 *Original papers*

Armstrong, C.M. (1969). Inactivation of the potassium conductance and related phenomena caused by quaternary ammonium ion injection in squid axons. *J. Gen. Physiol.* **54**, 553–575.

Armstrong, C. and Bezanilla, F. (1977). Inactivation of the sodium channel II. Gating current experiments. *J. Gen. Physiol.* **70**, 567–590.

Doyle, D.A. *et al.* (1998). The structure of the potassium channel: molecular basis of K^+ conduction and selectivity. *Science*, **280**, 69–77.

Gellens, M.E. *et al.* (1992). Primary structure and functional expression of the human cardiac, voltage-dependent sodium channel. *Proc. Natl. Acad. Sci. USA* **89**, 554–558.

Hagiwara, S., Chichibu, S. and Naka, K.I. (1964). The effects of various ions on resting and spike potentials of barnacle muscle fibers. *J. Gen. Physiol.* **48**, 163–179.

Hamill, O.P. *et al.* (1981). Improved patch-clamp techniques for high-resolution current recording from cells and cell-free membrane patches. *Pflugers Arch.* **391**, 85–100.

Hille, B. (1967). The selective inhibition of delayed potassium currents in nerve by tetraethylammonium ion. *J. Gen. Physiol.* **50**, 1287–1302.
Hille, B. (1970). Ionic channels in nerve membranes. *Prog. Biophys. Mol. Biol.* **21**, 1–22.

Hodgkin, A.L. and Keynes, R.D. (1955). The potassium permeability of a giant nerve fibre. *J. Physiol.* **128**, 61–88.

Hoshi, T., Zagotta, W.N. and Aldrich, R.W. (1990). Biophysical and molecular mechanisms of Shaker potassium channel inactivation. *Science* **250**, 533–538.

Jiang, Y. *et al.* (2003). The principle of gating charge movement in a voltage-dependent K^+ channel. *Nature* **423**, 42–48.

Lenaeus, M.J., Vamvouka, M., Focia, P.F. and Gross, A. (2005). Structural basis of TEA blockade in a model potassium channel. *Nature Struct. Mol. Biol.* **12**, 454–459.

Lipkind, G.M. and Fozzard, H.A. (2000). KcsA crystal structure as framework for a molecular model of the Na channel pore. *Biochemistry* **40**, 6786–6794.

Lipkind, G.M. and Fozzard, H.A. (2008). Voltage-gated Na channel selectivity: the role of the conserved domain III lysine residue. *J. Gen. Physiol.* **131**, 523–529

Long, S.B., Campbell, E.B. and MacKinnon, R. (2005). Crystal structure of a mammalian voltage-dependent Shaker family K$^+$ channel. *Science* **309**, 897–903.

Narahashi, T., Moore, J.W. and Scott, W.R. (1964). Tetrodotoxin blockage of sodium conductance increase in lobster giant axons. *J. Gen. Physiol.* **47**, 965–974.

Narahashi, T., Anderson, N.C. and Moore, J.W. (1966). Tetrodotoxin does not block excitation from inside the nerve membrane. *Science.* **153**, 765–767.

Noda, M. *et al.* (1984). Primary structure of *Electrophorus electricus* sodium channel deduced from cDNA sequence. *Nature* **312**, 121–127.

Payandeh, J., Scheuer, T., Zheng, N. and Catterall, W.A. (2011). The crystal structure of a voltage-gated sodium channel. *Nature* **475**, 353–358

Sigel, E. (1990). The use of Xenopus oocytes for the functional expression of plasma membrane proteins. *J. Membrane Biol.* **117**, 201–221.

Tombola, F., Pathak, M.M. and Isacoff, E.Y. (2005). Voltage-sensing arginines in a potassium channel permeate and occlude cation-selective pores. *Neuron* **45**, 379–388

Trimmer, J.S. *et al.* (1989). Primary structure and functional expression of a mammalian skeletal muscle sodium channel. *Neuron* **3**, 33–49.

Zagotta, W.N., Hoshi, T. and Aldrich, R.W. (1990). Restoration of inactivation in mutants of Shaker potassium channels by a peptide derived from ShB. *Science* **250**, 568–571.

Chapter 5

Active Transporters

We have learnt from previous chapters that channel opening allows a particular ion to diffuse across the membrane according to its electrochemical gradient. If this ion movement is not counteracted in some way, the concentration differences across the cell membrane will slowly dissipate and cell excitability will gradually be lost. Cells maintain the chemical gradients upon which the ionic movement depends by using another group of membrane transport proteins known collectively as active transporters.

5.1 Chapter objectives

After reading this chapter you should be able to:
- List and compare the properties of active transporters with those of channels
- Describe the structure and function of the Na^+/K^+ ATPase, the Na^+/Ca^{2+} exchanger and the Na^+/H^+ exchanger
- Discuss how the intracellular concentrations of Na^+, H^+ and Ca^{2+} are regulated and why the concentration of one of these ions plays a role in determining the concentration of the others

5.2 What do active transporters do?

These proteins move ions (and some amino acids and sugars) against their electrochemical gradients by forming complexes with them and then changing their conformation to deliver the ion on the other side of the membrane. The processes of ion binding, conformational switching and then unbinding are much slower than moving an ion through a channel. There are different types of active transporter largely categorized on whether or not they use ATP as an energy source.

To move ions against their concentration gradient requires some form of energy input. Some transporters use the energy derived from the hydrolysis of ATP and these are called ATPases or pumps. Other transporters do not use ATP but, instead, use the large electrochemical gradients of some ions as an energy source. The movement of one ion *against* its concentration (and/or electrical) gradient is coupled to the transport of another ion *down* its gradient resulting in an exchange of ionic species across the membrane. Such transporters are therefore termed ion exchangers.

General properties of channels
- Channels show gating
- Channels move ions rapidly (tens of millions of ions per channel per second)
- Ion movement always results in net charge movement

General properties of active transporters
- Active transporters do not show gating
- Active transporters move ions less rapidly (hundreds of ions per transporter per second)
- May be electroneutral or electrogenic
- Pumps or ATPases use ATP to move ions
- Exchangers generally do not require ATP as an energy source

5.3   ATPases or pumps

In the heart, important ATPases are the sodium–potassium pump (or Na^+/K^+-ATPase) and the calcium pump (Ca^{2+}-ATPase), one form of which exists in the sarcoplasmic reticulum membrane and another in the surface membrane. They belong to a group of proteins known as P-type ATPases (or E1-E2 ATPases), so-called because they catalyze the auto-phosphorylation of a common aspartate residue and cycle through two different conformations, E1 and E2, when transporting the ions.

5.3.1 *Na$^+$/K$^+$-ATPase*

In Chapter 2 we explained how the membrane potential arose as a result of the concentration of K$^+$ being typically about 20 to 30 times greater inside cells compared with its extracellular concentration. The opposite situation applies to Na$^+$, which has a low intracellular concentration compared with its concentration outside the cell. The concentration differences are maintained by Na$^+$/K$^+$ pumps located in the surface membranes of the cells. Discovery of the Na$^+$/K$^+$ pump can be attributed to a Danish scientist, Jens Christian Skou, who, in the 1950s, described the effects of Na$^+$ and K$^+$ on the hydrolysis of ATP in membrane fractions of crab nerves. He jointly received the Nobel Prize in Chemistry in 1997 for the discovery. The pumps extrude Na$^+$ ions from the cell cytoplasm whilst pumping K$^+$ ions from the extracellular fluid into the cell. Both ions are pumped against their concentration gradients using the energy derived from the hydrolysis of ATP. The pumping cycle, pictorially represented in Fig. 5.1, can be summarized as follows:

1   The pump is in a conformation called E1 when three Na$^+$ ions bind into a pocket in the trans-membrane domain of the protein from the cytoplasmic entryway. The exit pathway remains closed.

2   The enzyme catalyses its own phosphorylation by ATP at a conserved aspartate (Asp) residue which shuts the cytoplasmic entryway.

3   Following the release of ADP to the cytoplasm the conformation of the protein then changes to E2, which results in the extracellular exit path opening and a decrease in the affinity for the three Na$^+$ ions nestling within the protein. These are then released to the extracellular side.

4   Two K$^+$ ions from the extracellular side bind to the pump which is still in conformation E2.

5   The binding of the K$^+$ ions leads to the closure of the extracellular entryway and dephosphorylation and the protein returns to conformation E1.

6   With the return to E1, the affinity of the pump for Na$^+$ ions is restored and that for the counter ions reduced, ATP binding occurs and the two K$^+$ ions are released into the cytoplasm.

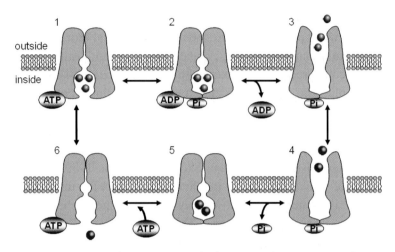

Figure 5.1. The pumping cycle of the Na$^+$/K$^+$ pump. Na$^+$ ions in blue, K$^+$ ions in red. See text for details.

The pumping process has a stoichiometry of 3:2; i.e. in one complete cycle three Na$^+$ ions are moved out of the cell and two K$^+$ ions are moved in, and so the net effect of a complete cycle of the pump is to move one positive charge out of the cell creating a pump current (I_p). The pump is therefore termed "electrogenic". In physiological circumstances it produces an outward current that helps to hyperpolarize the cell and makes a small contribution to the overall membrane potential, as outlined in Chapter 2. At any one membrane potential, the size of the pump current is dependent upon the intracellular [Na$^+$]. Estimates of the intracellular [Na$^+$] required to produce half-maximal I_p vary according to the experimental conditions used, but in the presence of physiological values of extracellular [Na$^+$] it is around 10–15 mM (rising with typical Michaelis–Menten saturation kinetics to near maximum pump current being observed at about 50 mM Na$^+$). Since intracellular [Na$^+$] is about 10 mM, this K_m value means the pump is tuned to responding to changes in [Na$^+$] and regulating the intracellular levels of the ion. The pump current is also dependent on extracellular [K$^+$] with the half-maximal I_p being about 1.5 mM and near maximum pump current being produced between 5 and 10 mM. Since serum potassium levels are between 3.5 and 5 mM the pump is about 80–90% saturated with K$^+$ ions under normal physiological conditions. This means that pump function is dictated almost exclusively by the intracellular [Na$^+$].

The current density (the amount of current flowing through a specific area of membrane) of the Na$^+$/K$^+$ pump is about 1 μA.cm^{-2} (or 1 A.F^{-1} – assuming specific membrane capacitance is 1 μF.cm^{-2}). Assuming also that a net single charge (1.6 $\times$ 10^{-19} C) is transferred per pump then the pump site density is around 2 200 to 2 800 pumps.μm^{-2} for ventricular cells. Contrast this with there being about 10–12 Na$^+$ channels.μm^{-2} on the surface membrane of ventricular cells.

It is obvious that I_p is also dependent on intracellular [ATP]. Half-maximal current is experimentally achieved with an [ATP] around 150 μM and, since intracellular [ATP] under physiological conditions is several millimolar, pump function is not usually compromised.

Rather analogous to the reversal potential of an ionic current flowing through a channel, the pump also has a reversal potential. With physiological concentrations of the ions E_{rev} is about −180 mV, which makes analysis of what happens when this potential is reached largely irrelevant. E_{rev} becomes less negative when the intracellular [ATP] falls and so pump direction may change when the cells become hypoxic or ischaemic, but this situation would only be encountered pathologically.

The Na$^+$/K$^+$ pump comprises three subunits, α, β and γ, as illustrated in Fig. 5.2. The α-subunit is the largest of the three at around 110 kDa and is structurally similar to the Ca^{2+}-ATPase in the sarcoplasmic reticulum. (The dalton (Da) is the standard unit used for indicating atomic mass and is equivalent to 1 g.mol^{-1}.) The α-subunit contains the sequences of amino acids that form the catalytic and ion-binding sites so is responsible for the main pump function. It is the pharmacological receptor for inhibitors such as digoxin and ouabain which bind when the pump is in its E2-P state, just after K$^+$ ions enter from the extracellular side. It is thought that the binding of these compounds inhibits the closure of the extracellular entryway.

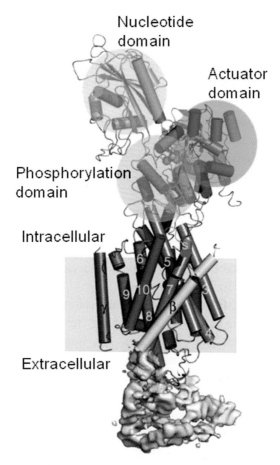

Figure 5.2.   The three-dimensional structure of the Na⁺/K⁺ pump. The grey area represents the cell membrane. Above this lies the cytoplasm and below the extracellular space. The α-subunit structures are shaded in blue with various trans-membrane domains numbered in yellow starting from the N-terminal of the molecule.   The β-subunit is shaded in mauve and extends out of the membrane into the extracellular space where its structure is represented by an electron density map. The γ-subunit is coloured in red. The main three cytoplasmic domains are shown coloured green (phosphorylation), blue (actuator) and orange (nucleotide). From Morth *et al.* (2007) *Nature* **450**, 1043–1049.

The α-subunit is composed of ten trans-membrane α-helices (usually denoted M1–M10). Additionally, there are three functional domains located on the cytoplasmic face of the membrane: the actuator domain

(A), the nucleotide-binding domain (N), and the phosphorylation domain (P). ATP binds to the nucleotide domain with resultant phosphorylation of the phosphorylation domain. The actuator domain couples this reaction to the conformational change that opens the occlusion site for sodium or potassium binding, depending whether the protein is in state E1 or E2. M4 contains the proline–glutamic acid–glycine–leucine (PEGL) signature motif of P-type ATPases and in association with M5 and M6 makes up the area in which the ions bind and are transported. M7 and M10 are involved in binding the β-subunit. The C-terminal of the α-subunit regulates the affinity of the ion coordination sites. It inhibits kinking of the molecule around the Gly 855 residue, which alters the configuration of the ion-binding site favouring sodium binding.

The β-subunit is smaller than the α-subunit with a molecular weight of about 53 kDa, and regulates the transport of pumps to the plasma membrane and conformational changes to the protein during the translocation of K^+. Much of the β-subunit lies on the extracellular side of the cell membrane acting as a lid for the K^+ and Na^+ coordination sites.

The γ-subunit is not required for pump function – the α- and β-subunits alone produce a fully functional protein. The γ-subunit is an accessory regulatory protein comprising a trans-membrane α-helix and an extracellular domain and is one of the "FXYD" family of proteins. These are small membrane proteins that share a 35-amino acid signature sequence domain, beginning with the sequence PFXYD (proline–phenylalanine–X–tyrosine–aspartate, with X often another tyrosine). FXYD1 is the γ-subunit of the Na^+/K^+ pump in the heart. It is also known as phospholemman and the extent of its phosphorylation determines pump activity.

5.3.2 *Na^+/K^+ pump isoforms*

The α-subunit has four isoforms, α1, α2, α3 and α4. The α4-isoform appears to be only expressed in sperm and is specifically synthesized for sperm motility. There are three isoforms of the β-subunit: β1, β2 and β3.

Most cells in the body express α1 and one of the other isoforms, all of which have different kinetic properties. The α1 has the highest affinity for Na$^+$ (as already noted to be about 10 mM). The α2- and α3-isoforms have apparent K_m's of about 20–30 mM – the K_m increasing in sequence α1 < α2 < α3. Assuming Na$^+$ fluxes do not change, these differences in affinities for Na$^+$ would mean that cells expressing mostly α2 or α3 would tend to have a higher resting intracellular [Na$^+$] compared with those predominantly expressing α1. In human heart α1, α2 and α3 are expressed together with β1. β2 is only expressed at very low levels. The distribution of the isoforms is variable over different areas of the heart and there is a good deal of speculation about the functional outcome of this variable distribution. There is also controversy regarding whether there is a sub-cellular differential distribution of isoforms. The consequences for this being the case are quite profound. If there are areas of the cells (say T-tubules) to which certain isoforms are localized, this may mean there are sub-cellular gradients of [Na$^+$]. As we will see, intracellular [Na$^+$] plays a major role in regulating the function of another active transporter, the Na$^+$/Ca^{2+} exchange. This transporter helps regulate Ca^{2+} levels in the cell so local gradients of [Na$^+$] may give rise to sub-cellular "microdomains" with different [Ca^{2+}] and, since this ion has significant cell signalling functions, subtle sub-cellular differences in ion homeostasis and cell biochemistry may result.

The α1-isoform has at least 300 times lower affinity for the pump inhibitor, ouabain, compared with the other isoforms. There is evidence for an endogenous circulating ouabain, most likely secreted from the adrenal gland, which may regulate cell Ca^{2+} signalling by inhibiting only α2 or α3 in the heart and perhaps controlling the microdomain [Na$^+$].

5.3.3   *Na$^+$/K$^+$ pump current and intracellular [Na$^+$]*

Figure 5.3 illustrates how membrane potential and pump current change during and after pump inhibition. In both cases the pump has been inhibited by removing extracellular [K$^+$]. When the preparation is not voltage clamped, pump inhibition produces a depolarization predicted because the pump current is outward and makes some contribution to

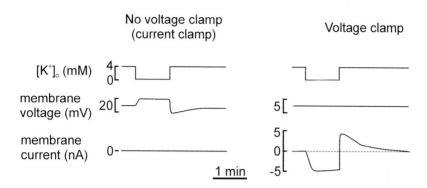

Figure 5.3. The figure illustrates the effect of inhibiting the Na⁺/K⁺ pumps in a dog Purkinje fibre. In the left panel the preparation is not voltage clamped. Pump inhibition by removing extracellular K⁺ ions produces a depolarization. The right panel shows the current changes in the same preparation when it is voltage clamped. Inhibiting the pump produces an inward change in the holding current. Adapted from Gadsby and Cranefield (1979) *Proc. Nat. Acad. Sci. USA* **76**, 1783–1787.

membrane potential. When the pump is re-stimulated (by adding back K⁺) there is a transient hyperpolarization that gradually declines to the resting membrane potential. The same experimental manoeuvres are then done when the preparation is voltage clamped. Pump inhibition produces a change in holding current that is inward (negative) because its outward current contribution has been removed and the consequent effect of this is measured. When the pump is re-stimulated, membrane current overshoots transiently in the outward direction then decays to the steady-state holding current.

The underlying reason for these changes in potential and current is the change in intracellular [Na⁺] that is taking place during pump inhibition. Figure 5.4 shows the change in intracellular [Na⁺] during a similar series of experimental manoeuvres. Pump inhibition produces an increase in intracellular [Na⁺] above normal steady-state levels. When the pump is re-started, membrane current overshoots transiently in the outward direction because it is stimulated by the increased intracellular [Na⁺]. The decay of the pump current to a steady state reflects the expulsion of Na⁺.

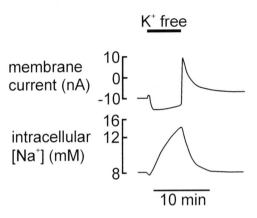

Figure 5.4. The figure illustrates the effect on intracellular [Na$^+$] of inhibiting the Na$^+$/K$^+$ pumps in a sheep Purkinje fibre.   Pump inhibition by removing extracellular K$^+$ ions produces an inward change in the holding current and the intracellular [Na$^+$] (note the logarithmic scale) starts to increase. Adapted from Eisner *et al.* (1981) *J. Physiol.* **317**, 163–187.

5.4 Ion exchangers

Other types of transporters couple the movement of one ion against its concentration (and/or electrical) gradient to the transport of another ion down its gradient resulting in an exchange of ionic species. ATP is not consumed; instead, energy is derived from the electrochemical gradient. A typical ion exchanger and one that is essential for the control of intracellular Ca^{2+} in the heart is the sarcolemmal sodium–calcium exchanger (Na$^+$/Ca^{2+} exchanger, or NCX). It uses the large electrochemical gradient for Na$^+$ ions entering the cell to provide the necessary energy to expel Ca^{2+} ions from the cell against their electrochemical gradient.

5.4.1 *Na$^+$/Ca^{2+} exchanger*

The observation that there was a coupled exchange of Na$^+$ and Ca^{2+} across cell membranes was first made in heart muscle by Reuter and Seitz in 1968 although the importance of extracellular [Na$^+$] on cardiac contraction had been noted in 1921 by de Burgh Daly and Clark. They wrote:

> The effect of reducing the NaCl content of Ringer to one-half was to improve the general activity of the heart... When the NaCl content was reduced to a quarter the heart passed into a condition of semi-systole... When a fluid containing no sodium chloride was perfused, the heart immediately contracted into systole...

We will learn the underlying reasons for these observations later. The primary "beat-to-beat" function of the exchange in heart cells is to remove an amount of Ca^{2+} from the cytoplasm equivalent to that which enters the cell during the action potential to trigger contraction, thereby keeping the cell in Ca^{2+} balance. Like the Na^+/K^+ pump, NCX is also electrogenic but with a stoichiometry of 3:1. Three Na^+ ions are transported into the cell in exchange for one Ca^{2+} ion expelled, so one net positive charge enters for every Ca^{2+} ion that is removed producing a current (I_{NCX}). This Na^+ influx/Ca^{2+} efflux direction is designated as the "forward mode" of the exchanger. Under some conditions the exchanger can work in so-called "reverse mode" linking Na^+ efflux with Ca^{2+} influx. Ultimately the direction is governed by the electrochemical gradients of each ion. The energy required to expel a Ca^{2+} ion will be equivalent to its driving force times its charge, i.e. $(E_{Ca} - E_m)zF$ (where E_{Ca} is the equilibrium potential for Ca^{2+} calculated as described in Chapter 2). At equilibrium the amount of electrochemical driving force supplied by the Na^+ gradient will balance that required for the efflux of Ca^{2+}, so for a stoichiometry of 3:1 then:

$$3(E_{Na} - E_m)zF = (E_{Ca} - E_m)zF \qquad (5.1)$$

The direction of ion movement will vary with membrane potential and will reverse at E_{rev}:

$$E_{rev} = 3E_{Na} - 2E_{Ca} \qquad (5.2)$$

At this point there will be no net ion movement and, at membrane potentials more positive than the reversal potential, the exchanger will carry Ca^{2+} into the cell and Na^+ will be expelled. Under normal resting

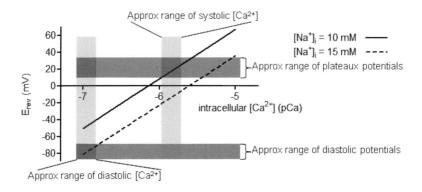

Figure 5.5. E_{rev} plotted as a function of intracellular $[Ca^{2+}]$. At membrane potentials more negative than E_{rev} the exchange will work in Na^+ influx/Ca^{2+} efflux (forward) mode. At membrane potentials more positive than E_{rev} the exchange will work in Na^+ efflux/Ca^{2+} influx (reverse) mode.

conditions when the heart cells are quiescent and intracellular $[Ca^{2+}]$ is low (around 100 nM), E_{rev} is about –50 mV but becomes more positive when the cytoplasmic $[Ca^{2+}]$ increases rapidly on excitation. Figure 5.5 shows the reversal potential plotted as a function of the intracellular $[Ca^{2+}]$. This illustrates the point that E_{rev} changes as intracellular $[Ca^{2+}]$ increases and decreases during the contraction and relaxation cycles of the heart muscle cells. E_{rev} is also dependent upon intracellular $[Na^+]$ and if this increases Fig. 5.5 shows that E_{rev} becomes more negative. Therefore, whether the exchange works in its forward or reverse mode is determined by the membrane potential of the cell, the intracellular $[Na^+]$ and intracellular $[Ca^{2+}]$, and these all change during the cardiac cycle.

I_{NCX} will normally be inward when the exchange performs its primary function but the current can become outward depending on how the above determinants alter. Figure 5.6 illustrates how the function of the exchanger changes during the action potential. In Panel A the action potential from a ventricular cell (top trace), the corresponding Ca^{2+} transient (middle trace) and the Na^+/Ca^{2+} exchange current (bottom trace) are plotted when intracellular $[Na^+]$ is 10 mM. Notice that I_{NCX} is

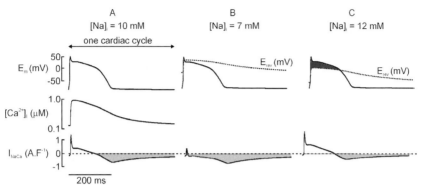

Figure 5.6.   The function of NCX during the action potential. Panel A: (top) action potential from a ventricular cell, (middle) the corresponding Ca^{2+} transient and (bottom) the Na^+/Ca^{2+} exchange current when intracellular $[Na^+]$ is 10 mM. Light grey shaded area denotes inward I_{NCX}. Panel B: similar conditions as A except the cell has an intracellular $[Na^+]$ of 7 mM. E_{rev} of the exchange (dotted line) superimposed on the action potential during the whole cardiac cycle. Panel C: similar conditions as A except the cell has an intracellular $[Na^+]$ of 12 mM. Dark grey shaded area denotes time NCX is in outward (or reverse) mode. Adapted from Bers (1987) *J. Gen. Physiol.* **90**, 479–504.

outward at the start of the action potential but as the plateau terminates it becomes inward and remains in the forward mode for the rest of the cardiac cycle, as denoted by the light grey shaded area. Panel B illustrates how I_{NCX} changes when all the conditions are exactly the same during the cardiac cycle as in Panel A except the cell has an intracellular $[Na^+]$ of 7 mM instead of 10 mM. I_{NCX} is only outward for a very brief period at the start of the action potential and for most of the cardiac cycle is inward (again note the difference in time occupied by the light grey shaded area).

Superimposed on the action potential is E_{rev} plotted during the whole cycle. Only when membrane potential becomes more positive than E_{rev} will the exchanger work in outward (or reverse) mode. The tiny dark grey shaded area illustrates when this happens. In Panel C again all the conditions are exactly the same during the cardiac cycle as in Panel A except the cell has an intracellular $[Na^+]$ of 12 mM. In this condition I_{NCX} spends a longer portion of the cardiac cycle in the reverse mode and proportionately less in the forward mode. Compare the trace of E_{rev} superimposed on the action potential. The membrane potential is more positive than E_{rev} for a much longer time, as shown by the dark grey shaded area.

NCX is a member of a family of three similar exchanger proteins (NCX 1, 2 and 3) that are widely expressed and share considerable amino acid homology. NCX 1 is the cardiac isoform but is itself widely expressed in various other tissues. NCX 1 is composed of 970 amino acids and has a molecular weight of 110 kDa. The amino acids form nine trans-membrane segments (TMS), a large intracellular loop between TMS 5–6 and two re-entrant loops (a re-entrant loop is a structure that goes about half-way through the membrane then turns back to the side from which it originates) connecting TMS 2–3 and TMS 7–8 (Fig. 5.7). The re-entrant loops are involved in Na^+ and Ca^{2+} ion binding and transport and the large intracellular loop is concerned with exchange regulation. The binding of Ca^{2+} to sites on the large loop modulates and activates the exchange, so intracellular Ca^{2+} is both a substrate that is transported and an activating ligand. Removal of the loop still produces an active exchanger. Protein kinase A and C phosphorylation sites have also been identified on the cytoplasmic loop. Stimulation of β-adrenergic receptors increases NCX activity via PKA-mediated phosphorylation as does PKC-mediated phosphorylation via an α-adrenoceptor signalling pathway.

Although a considerable body of work describing NCX structure and function exists, the precise nature and location of the ion translocation pathway is still unclear. However, the crystal structure of the transport section of the protein has very recently been established in a homologue of NCX isolated from *Methanococcus jannaschii* (an organism found in extreme environments such as at the bottom of some oceans surrounded by water at high temperature and pressure) at 1.9 Å resolution. This form of the protein has no large intracellular regulatory loop and has ten trans-membrane domains instead of nine, but closely resembles the basic functional unit of isoforms of NCX. Investigation of its structure at this resolution has produced the following preliminary picture of how the molecule transports Na^+ and Ca^{2+}.

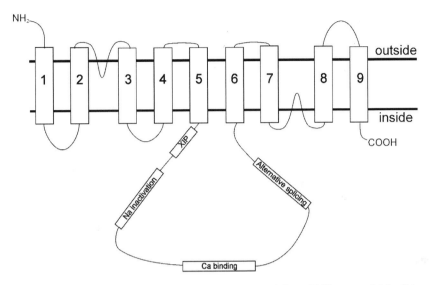

Figure 5.7.   Diagram of the structure of NCX.   Adapted from Philipson and Nicoll (2000) *Ann. Rev. Physiol.* **62**,111–133.

When the exchange protein is in the confirmation whereby both entrance passages are facing extracellularly, the large concentration of Na^+ causes entry of these ions into the molecule and the occupation the Na^+ binding sites (Fig. 5.8). It appears that there are four ion-binding sites grouped near each other towards the centre of the protein,   one relatively specific for Ca^{2+} and three with affinities appropriate for binding Na^+ ions at physiologically relevant concentrations.   Access to these binding sites is provided by two passageways from the same side of the protein. Although the Ca^{2+}-specific site can be reached from both sides of the molecule, the Na^+ sites are aligned in a single file along the passageway and can only be reached from one side of the molecule. Whether this side is facing externally or towards the cytoplasm will dictate the mode of transport for the exchange.

The binding of Na^+ decreases the affinity of the Ca^{2+} binding site causing release of Ca^{2+} to the extracellular space and so the exchange reaction occurs. The molecule undergoes a conformational change so that the entry/exit passageways face intracellularly. The three bound Na^+ ions

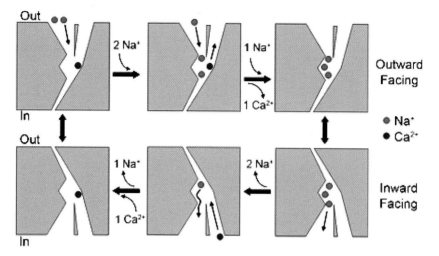

Figure 5.8.   A proposed sequence of Na$^+$/Ca^{2+} exchange operation based on knowledge of the crystal structure of the protein. With permission from Liao *et al.* (2012) *Science* **335**, 686–690.

are now exposed to an environment much lower in [Na$^+$] and start to unbind. The release of Na$^+$ restores the higher affinity form of the Ca^{2+} binding site which then binds Ca^{2+} again and another conformational change resets the molecule to an extracellular-facing form.

5.4.2 *Na$^+$/H$^+$ exchanger*

Another important active transporter in cardiac muscle is the Na$^+$/H$^+$ exchanger (or NHE). Again the gradient of Na$^+$, produced by the Na$^+$/K$^+$ pump, provides the necessary driving force for H$^+$ ion extrusion with a stoichiometry of 1:1. The electroneutral exchange performs an important role in regulating intracellular pH, an important parameter in the heart because muscle contraction is very sensitive to pH. If we make a calculation of the expected intracellular pH if protons were in equilibrium across the cell membrane it would be near to 6.2 but the measured intracellular pH is about 7.2, an order of magnitude more alkali. There must be active mechanisms maintaining this proton gradient and one of these is the Na$^+$/H$^+$ exchanger. The exchanger is activated as

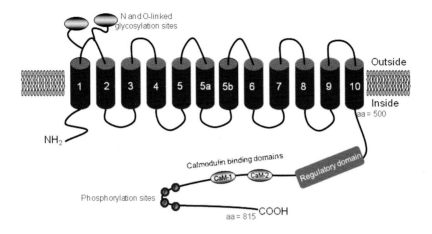

Figure 5.9.   Diagram of the structure of the Na^+/H^+ exchange.

intracellular pH becomes more acid. H^+ ion flux through the exchanger is about ten times greater when intracellular pH is 6.7 compared with the flux when intracellular pH is 7.2. Nine isoforms of NHE have been described so far: NHE-1 to NHE-9. NHE-1 was the first isoform to be cloned. It is widely expressed in many tissues but is considered to be the cardiac-specific isoform.

NHE-1 comprises 815 amino acids and has a predicted molecular mass of about 91 kDa, but because the protein is glycosylated its molecular mass is nearer 110 kDa. It has two quite distinct functional domains: an N-terminal region of about 500 amino acids with 12 trans-membrane areas and a cytoplasmic regulatory C-terminal region of about 300 amino acids in length. The former is involved in ion translocation and inhibitor binding and includes the H^+ sensing site that promotes activation of the exchange as intracellular pH becomes more acid, whilst the latter encompasses the regulatory sites modulating the function of the exchange by phosphorylation reactions as well as another H^+ sensing site (see Fig. 5.9).

NHE-1 is not the only mechanism protecting cardiac cells from acidosis. Based on experiments demonstrating HCO_3^- -dependent acid recovery of intracellular pH that was not affected by the NHE-1 inhibitor amiloride, another type of active transporter exists. This is a co-transporter (sometimes called a symporter) using the energy gradient of Na^+ to transport HCO_3^- *into* cells. It is called the Na^+/HCO_3^- symport and its stoichiometry is probably 1:1, so it is electroneutral and mediates net acid extrusion.

5.5   Interaction of ion transporters in the heart

Individually these particular transporters ensure homeostatic control of intracellular Na^+, Ca^{2+} and pH but the regulation of one ion is linked very closely to that of the others and they all have modulatory influences on cardiac contraction.

5.5.1   *The effect of alterations to intracellular [Na⁺] on contractile force*

There is a close quantitative relation between intracellular $[Na^+]$ and contractile force. Consider the experiment on voltage-clamped cardiac Purkinje fibres illustrated in Fig. 5.10. In this experiment, the Na^+ pump was inhibited with strophanthidin (an analogue of ouabain) and the preparation clamped regularly to depolarizing potentials to produce contraction. Notice that as intracellular $[Na^+]$ increased so did contractile force. There is a steep relation between contraction and intracellular $[Na^+]$. This is because an increase in intracellular $[Na^+]$ will cause the reversal potential for the Na^+/Ca^{2+} exchange to become more negative.

During the action potential the exchange will then spend more time in the reverse mode than under normal intracellular $[Na^+]$ (see Fig. 5.6) so this will push the exchange to more Ca^{2+} influx and less Ca^{2+} efflux. Contraction is increased because of two factors. Firstly, increasing Ca^{2+} influx allows the sarcoplasmic reticulum to fill with more Ca^{2+} which will be available for release at the next beat. Secondly, the resting level of intracellular $[Ca^{2+}]$ will increase (with minimal effect on resting force)

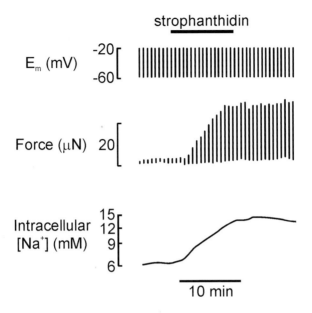

Figure 5.10. The effects of inhibiting the Na^+/K^+ pump with strophanthidin on force production and intracellular $[Na^+]$. Sheep heart Purkinje fibres were voltage clamped and depolarized from about -60 to -20 mV to produce contraction. Adapted from Eisner *et al.* (1983) *J. Physiol.* **335**, 723–743.

so that the same increment in Ca^{2+} released from the sarcoplasmic reticulum will produce greater force because of the sigmoidal nature of the relation between intracellular $[Ca^{2+}]$ and force.

This is the mechanism by which cardiac glycosides and steroids are believed to work. These compounds inhibit the Na^+/K^+ pump which leads to an increase in intracellular $[Na^+]$. The increase in intracellular $[Na^+]$ pushes the exchange to more Ca^{2+} influx and less Ca^{2+} efflux during the cycle; intracellular $[Ca^{2+}]$ increases and so contraction becomes more powerful.

5.5.2 *The effect of alterations to intracellular pH on contractile force*

The effects of acid and alkali solutions on the heart had been appreciated since the laboratory work by William Gaskell MD in 1880. He noted,

> When, by means of an acid solution, the beats of the ventricle have been very much lowered in force, then the alkaline solution brings back the force of the beat to its original height, and then produces its own characteristic effect, ... the beats are strengthened.

We know today that the effects Gaskell observed are mainly due to changes in intracellular pH occurring as a result of alterations in extracellular pH. Probably the largest effect of intracellular pH on contraction is brought about through modifications in the binding of Ca^{2+} to the troponin complex, the regulatory myofibrillar protein. In acidotic conditions there is a decrease in the affinity of troponin C for Ca^{2+} that leads to a decrease in cross-bridge formation and so active force production (see Fig. 5.11). Increasing intracellular pH from 7.0 to 7.4 shifts the force versus $[Ca^{2+}]$ relationship to the left so that a lower cytoplasmic $[Ca^{2+}]$ is required to obtain the same force, decreases the threshold $[Ca^{2+}]$ required for contraction and increases the maximum force that can be obtained in the presence of saturating $[Ca^{2+}]$. Changes of intracellular pH in the acid direction produce opposite results.

Therefore, intracellular $[Na^+]$ and pH both influence the strength of contraction and though their relative levels are controlled by separate mechanisms the two are closely related because of interactions between H^+ and Ca^{2+}.

5.5.3 *Interactions between H^+ and Ca^{2+}*

An early demonstration that changes in cytoplasmic $[Ca^{2+}]$ can alter the intracellular pH is illustrated below in Fig. 5.12. Injections of $CaCl_2$ into snail neurones acidified the cytoplasm and the degree of acidosis was dependent upon the amount of Ca^{2+} injected. Longer injections of $CaCl_2$ into snail neurones produced larger acidic departures in intracellular pH. In the heart, similar effects occur suggesting significant interaction

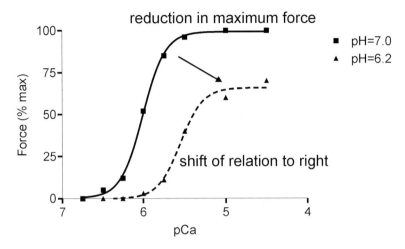

Figure 5.11. The effect of acidotic pH on the relation between pCa and force production in skinned cardiac muscle cells. Redrawn from Fabiato and Fabiato (1978) *J. Physiol.* **276**, 233–255.

between the intracellular buffering of H^+ and Ca^{2+}. The converse experiment, i.e. changing intracellular pH and measuring the effect on intracellular $[Ca^{2+}]$ produces similar evidence for interaction between H^+ and Ca^{2+}. As intracellular pH becomes more alkaline, intracellular $[Ca^{2+}]$ decreases and when intracellular pH falls, intracellular $[Ca^{2+}]$ increases.

The exact mechanisms underlying the intracellular interaction of the two ions remain uncertain but are probably multi-factorial. There may be H^+-activated release of Ca^{2+} from mitochondria and the two ions may share common cytoplasmic buffering sites.

So there are two routes whereby an acidosis might lead to an increase in intracellular $[Ca^{2+}]$: firstly, the sharing of common buffering sites means that these will bind H^+ and release Ca^{2+}; secondly, the acidosis will activate the Na^+/H^+ exchange and Na^+/HCO_3^- symport leading to an increase in intracellular $[Na^+]$ which pushes NCX to more Ca^{2+} influx and less Ca^{2+} efflux during the cardiac cycle.

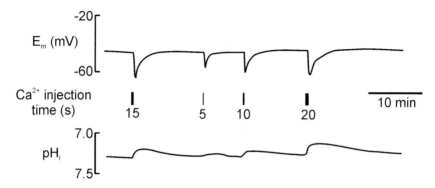

Figure 5.12.   The effect on intracellular pH (pH_i) of different amounts of Ca^{2+} ion injected into the cell. The amount of Ca^{2+} ion injected was varied by altering the time of injection. Redrawn from Meech and Thomas (1977) *J. Physiol.* **265**, 867–879.

5.6 Summary

- Channels show gating whereas active transporters do not. Active transporters move ions less rapidly than channels. Ion movement through channels always results in net charge movement whereas transporters may be electroneutral or electrogenic.
- The Na^+/K^+ pump is a P-type ATPase with a stoichiometry of 3:2. The intracellular $[Na^+]$ required to produce half-maximal pump current is between 10 and 15 mM. Since intracellular $[Na^+]$ is about 10 mM, this K_m value means the pump is tuned to responding to physiological changes in intracellular $[Na^+]$.
- The Na^+/K^+ pump comprises three subunits, α, β and γ. The α-subunit contains key functional domains. ATP binds to the nucleotide-binding domain with resultant phosphorylation of the P-domain. The A-domain couples this reaction to the conformational change that opens the occlusion site for sodium or potassium binding.
- The β-subunit of the Na^+/K^+ pump regulates the transport of newly synthesized pumps to the plasma membrane and the γ-subunit is not required for function but can modulate pump activity.

- The Na^+/Ca^{2+} exchange is electrogenic with a stoichiometry of 3:1. Three Na^+ ions are transported into the cell in exchange for one Ca^{2+} ion expelled; the gradient of Na^+ providing the necessary driving force for Ca^{2+} ion extrusion. This Na^+ influx/Ca^{2+} efflux direction is designated as the "forward mode". Under some conditions the exchanger can work in so-called "reverse mode" linking Na^+ efflux with Ca^{2+} influx. Transport direction is governed by the intracellular concentrations of Na^+ and Ca^{2+} and membrane potential.

- The Na^+/H^+ exchanger also uses the gradient of Na^+ to provide the driving force for H^+ ion extrusion with a stoichiometry of 1:1. The exchange performs an important role in regulating intracellular pH. H^+ ions are not in equilibrium across the cardiac cell membrane. Intracellular pH is about 7.2, an order of magnitude more alkali than if H^+ ions were passively distributed. The exchanger is activated as intracellular pH becomes more acid. NHE-1 is the main exchanger isoform in the heart.

- Intracellular interactions between Na^+, Ca^{2+} and H^+ are complex. There are two routes whereby increasing H^+ might lead to an increase in intracellular $[Ca^{2+}]$. The ions share common buffering sites and these will bind H^+ and release Ca^{2+}. The increase in concentration of H^+ will activate the Na^+/H^+ exchange and Na^+/HCO_3^- symport leading to an increase in intracellular $[Na^+]$, which pushes Na^+/Ca^{2+} exchange to more Ca^{2+} influx and less Ca^{2+} efflux during the cardiac cycle.

5.7 Questions

(1) Contrast the general properties of channels with those of active transporters.

(2) Calculate the reversal potential of the NCX given the following concentrations of Na^+ and Ca^{2+} extra- and intracellularly. $[Na^+]$ = 140 mM outside and 14 mM inside. $[Ca^{2+}]$ = 1.8 mM outside and 280 nM inside.

(3) Describe the mechanism by which cardiac glycosides and steroids are believed to work.

(4) Assuming $pH_i = 7.2$ and $pH_o = 7.4$ calculate E_H.

(5) Describe how an intracellular acidosis might lead to an increase in intracellular $[Ca^{2+}]$.

5.8 Bibliography

5.8.1 *Reviews*

Galougahi, K.K., Liu, C.C., Bundgaard. H. and Rasmussen, H.H. (2012). β-adrenergic regulation of the cardiac Na^+-K^+ ATPase mediated by oxidative signaling. *Trends Cardiovasc. Med.* **22**, 83–87.

Glitsch, H.G. (2001). Electrophysiology of the sodium-potassium-ATPase in cardiac cells. *Physiol. Rev.* **81**, 1791–1826.

Philipson, K.D. and Nicoll, D.A. (2000). Sodium-calcium exchange: a molecular perspective. *Ann. Rev. Physiol.* **62**, 111–133.

Sher, A.A., Noble, P.J., Hinch, R. *et al.* (2008). The role of the Na^+/Ca^{2+} exchangers in Ca^{2+} dynamics in ventricular myocytes. *Prog. Biophys. Mol. Biol.* **96**, 377–398.

Slepkov, E.R., Rainey, J.K., Sykes, B.D. and Fliegel, L. (2007). Structural and functional analysis of the Na^+/H^+ exchanger. *Biochem. J.* **401**, 623–633.

Vaughan-Jones, R.D., Villafuerte, F.C., Swietach, P. *et al.* (2006). pH-regulated Na^+ influx into the mammalian ventricular myocyte: the relative role of Na^+-H^+ exchange and Na^+-$HCO3^-$ co-transport. *J. Cardiovasc. Electrophysiol.* **17** Suppl. 1, S134–S140.

5.8.2 *Original papers*

de Burgh Daly, I. and Clark, A.J. (1921). The action of ions upon the frog's heart. *J. Physiol.* **54**, 367–383.

Bers, D.M. (1987). Mechanisms contributing to the cardiac inotropic effect of Na pump inhibition and reduction of extracellular Na. *J. Gen. Physiol.* **90**, 479–504.

Eisner, D.A., Lederer, W.J. and Vaughan-Jones, R.D. (1983). The control of tonic tension by membrane potential and intracellular sodium activity in sheep heart Purkinje fibres. *J. Physiol.* **335**, 723–743.

Fabiato, A. and Fabiato, F. (1978). Effects of pH on the myofilaments and the sarcoplasmic reticulum of skinned cells from cardiac and skeletal muscles. *J. Physiol.* **276**, 233–255.

Gadsby, D.C. and Cranefield, P.F. (1979). Direct measurement of changes in sodium pump current in canine cardiac Purkinje fibres. *Proc. Nat. Acad. Sci. USA.* **76**,1783–1787.

Gaskell, W.H. (1880). On the tonicity of the heart and blood vessels. *J. Physiol.* **3**, 48–75.

Liao, J., Zeng, W., Sauer, D.B. *et al.* (2012). Structural insight into the ion-exchange mechanism of the sodium/calcium exchanger. *Science* **335**, 686–690.

Meech, R.W. and Thomas, R.C. (1977). The effect of calcium injection on teh intracellular sodium and pH of snail neurones. *J. Physiol.* **265**, 867–879.

Morth, J.P., Pedersen, B.P., Toustrup-Jensen, M.S. *et al.* (2007). Crystal structure of the sodium–potassium pump. *Nature* **450**, 1043–1049.

Nakao, M. and Gadsby, D.C. (1989). [Na] and [K] dependence of the Na/K pump current-voltage relationship in guinea pig ventricular myocytes. *J. Gen. Physiol.* **94**, 539–565.

Reuter, H. and Seitz, N. (1968). The dependence of calcium efflux from cardiac muscle on temperature and external ion composition. *J. Physiol.* **195**, 451–470.

Skou, J.C. (1957). The influence of some cations on an adenosine triphosphatase from peripheral nerves. *Biochim. Biophys. Acta.* **23**, 394–401.

Chapter 6

Currents Flowing During the Early Part of the Ventricular Action Potential

In this chapter we will describe the important features of the early parts of the ventricular action potential and explain, in terms of the currents that flow during it, the underlying electrical events. The currents will be described as far as possible in the chronological order of their occurrence. In the next chapter we will move on to describing the currents flowing later in the ventricular action potential.

6.1 Chapter objectives

After reading this chapter you should be able to:

- Describe the different phases of the cardiac action potential
- Discuss how and over what range the Na^+ current activates
- Describe the mechanisms involved in Na^+ channel inactivation and how these determine refractory period
- Explain channel nomenclature
- Define early repolarization and discuss the role played by the transient outward current (I_{to}) in that process
- Discuss how and over what range $I_{Ca,L}$ operates
- Describe and illustrate using diagrams the role of $I_{Ca,L}$ in cardiac contraction
- Be familiar with Ca^{2+} channel structure
- Explain the mechanisms underlying L-type Ca^{2+} channel inactivation

- Discuss the various ways of modulating L-type Ca^{2+} channel function and the consequences of doing so.

6.2 Why describe the ventricular action potential?

There are a large number of different kinds of excitable cells in cardiac muscle. The contractile cells of the heart (cardiac myocytes) make up about 75 per cent of its mass whilst the other excitable myocytes are specialized for the initiation of the action potential (sino-atrial nodal cells) and its transmission (via cells of the atria, atrioventricular nodes, the bundle of His and Purkinje fibres) so that coordinated contraction of the four chambers occurs. This sequential excitation of the heart is the basis for the electrocardiogram. Each excitable cell type has a differently shaped action potential. The different action potential shapes are due to different ionic currents flowing that reflect different degrees of expression of ionic channels. For our purposes it is convenient at this point to confine our description of ionic currents to the main contractile cell in the heart – the ventricular myocyte – since this contains a large number of the more common currents flowing during the cardiac cycle and is well characterized.

6.3 The phases of the action potential

The ventricular action potential has a long duration compared with nerve (several hundred milliseconds versus a few milliseconds) and the time courses of the potential changes are very different. This is because the duration of the action potential controls the duration of contraction of the cell and a long, slow contraction is required to produce an effective pump. The long action potential also produces a long refractory period which, under normal circumstances, prevents the heart from contracting prematurely or contractions fusing (like tetanic contractions in skeletal muscle).

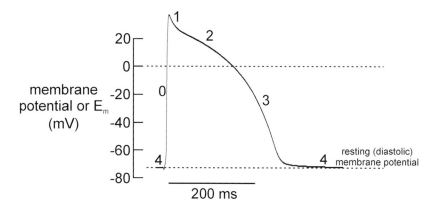

Figure 6.1. The phases of the cardiac action potential. Resting membrane potential in this cell is about –70 mV. The maximum potential reached during the upstroke (phase 0) is about +37 mV. The duration is around 300 ms.

A typical action potential from a ventricular cell is shown in Fig. 6.1 and it can be split into five phases:

Phase 0 – rapid upstroke characterized by a fast and large depolarization of the cell;

Phase 1 – early repolarization (aka "notch" or "spike") and contraction starts;

Phase 2 – plateau marks a period when the membrane potential is relatively stable then a prolonged phase of slow repolarization starts, contraction peaks and the cell begins relaxing;

Phase 3 – repolarization, which initially takes place slowly then more rapidly;

Phase 4 – resting membrane potential is reached.

6.4 Phase 4 – Resting membrane potential

We indicated in Chapter 2 that the ion that contributes most significantly to the resting membrane potential is K^+. Provided K^+ channels are open, K^+ ions will diffuse out of the cell down their concentration gradient and drive the membrane potential towards E_K. As we will see later, K^+ channels come in a variety of "flavours" in the ventricular myocyte membrane, but the K^+ current that is mainly responsible for forming the resting membrane potential is called I_{K1} and flows through a functionally distinct type of K^+-selective channel called the inward rectifying K^+ channel (K_{ir}). We will discuss these channels in more detail in the next chapter because their behaviour makes a major contribution to the prolonged plateau phase, the last part of the repolarization process and, needless to say, the resting membrane potential or phase 4. For the moment it is sufficient to state that the resting membrane potential is determined by the outward flow of K^+ ions through open K_{ir} channels together with a small contribution from the Na^+/K^+ pump. Both produce outward currents opposed by the much more limited permeabilities of other channels that create small inward "leak" fluxes of ions through some (randomly) open Na^+ and Ca^{2+} channels. Although at negative membrane potentials I_{K1} drives the membrane potential close to E_K, the inward leak current keeps that equilibrium potential from being reached.

6.5   Phase 0 – the rapid upstroke (Na^+ current)

The rapid depolarization of the cells producing the "upstroke" or phase 0 of the cardiac action potential is brought about by an increase in Na^+ channel conductance. Small depolarizations of neighbouring cells are sensed by the S4 and "voltage-sensor paddle" regions of the Na^+ channels (see Chapter 4). If the depolarizations are large enough (a so-called threshold value), the channel protein movements draw the S5 helices away from the pore, so inducing movement of S6 and the channels open. Once a small number of channels open, the probability of more channels opening becomes greater because the opening of these channels produces an inward flow of Na^+ ions that evoke a larger depolarization which, in turn, activates more channels. The result is a large increase in the open probability of the Na^+ channels culminating in the production of a large inward Na^+ current (I_{Na}).

I_{Na} activates over the voltage range shown in Fig. 6.2. At voltages more negative than –75 mV few channels activate, but as membrane potential becomes more positive more channels open with the relation becoming steep between –50 and –25 mV. Na^+ ions move into the cell

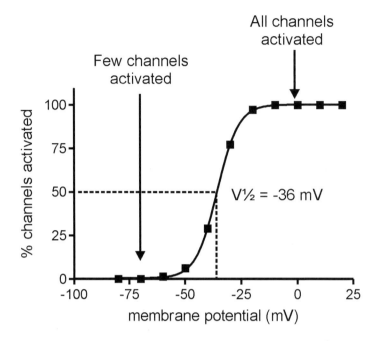

Figure 6.2. The voltage dependence of Na⁺ channel activation.

and drive (as discussed in Chapter 2), the trans-membrane potential towards E_{Na}, which results in the upstroke. This type of behaviour was observed in the squid axon by Hodgkin and Huxley.

Figure 6.3 shows how the Na⁺ current changes with the trans-membrane voltage. This relation has been obtained from a series of voltage clamp experiments of the type shown in Fig. 6.3A. The membrane potential of the cell has been clamped at −150 mV then stepped to the indicated test voltage as shown. The current obtained by each clamp step is shown plotted with respect to the clamp test potential in panel C. In the intact cell the Na⁺ current is maximal around −40 mV, reverses very near to the predicted E_{Na} value of +52 mV, is usually greater than 40 nA and peaks within 1 ms.

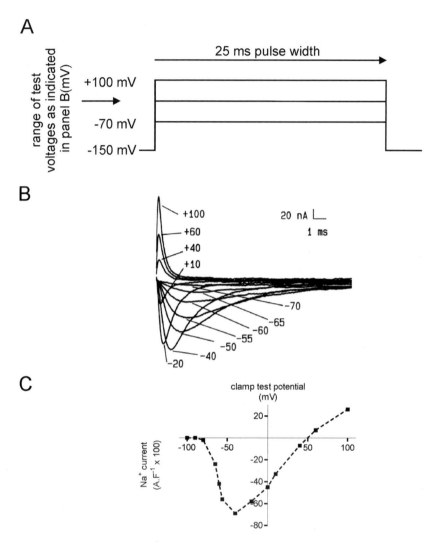

Figure 6.3. The effect of changing the membrane potential on Na^+ current (I_{Na}) in single canine Purkinje fibres. This experiment was carried out at room temperature with an extracellular and intracellular [Na^+] of 120 and 15 mM respectively. The cells were voltage clamped and held at -150 mV. They were then subjected to a series of test depolarizing clamp steps as indicated in Panel A. The currents evoked by the clamp steps from -150 mV are shown in Panel B and the resulting *I–V* relationship is plotted in Panel C. Current has been normalized to cell capacitance to account for variations in cell size, hence it is expressed in units $A.F^{-1}$. Redrawn from Makielski *et al.* (1987) *Biophys. J.* **52**, 1–11.

I_{Na} is the main current responsible for conduction of the excitatory wave through the ventricular walls. Its fast kinetics and high density impart rapid upstroke velocities (typically 200 $V.s^{-1}$ for ventricular myocardium) and brisk conduction (approximately 2 $m.s^{-1}$ for ventricular myocardium) of the action potential.

6.5.1 *Na^+ channel inactivation and refractory periods*

Just two milliseconds or so after the Na^+ channels open in response to membrane depolarization, they stop conducting ions despite the membrane still being depolarized.   The channels are now in an inactivated state. In Chapter 4 we described the existing views on the mechanisms underlying the process of inactivation. In Na^+ channels it appears to involve a loop of peptide linking the S3 and S4 domains that reacts to depolarization more slowly than the initial protein movements occurring on channel opening. It hinges to block the channel conduction pathway. Figure 6.4 shows the voltage dependency of Na^+ current inactivation (or Na^+ channel availability). As the membrane potential becomes more positive, channel availability decreases. Remember that inactivated Na^+ channels cannot be reactivated to their conducting state directly – the inactivation must be removed by repolarizing the membrane. This is the mechanism that underlies the absolute refractory period of an action potential. During this time no action potential can be initiated, regardless of the stimulus strength used (Fig. 6.5). Membrane repolarization must take place before the channels can conduct again so the channel will remain shut in the inactivated state until more negative potentials are reached, and this will not happen until the final phase (phase 3) of repolarization.

The absolute refractory period has a corollary in whole heart preparations called the effective refractory period. This is a period during which no propagating action potentials can be initiated no matter the stimulus strength. The relative refractory period follows the absolute period and is an interval during which an action potential can be elicited but the stimulus required is larger than normal (Fig. 6.5). It occurs as a result of the membrane repolarizing to a point where a portion of Na^+

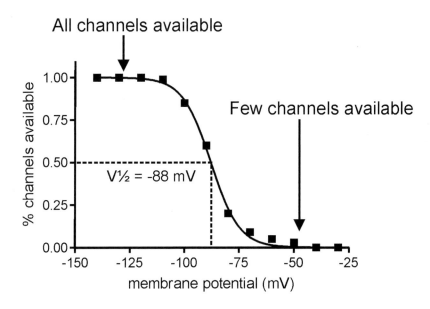

Figure 6.4. The voltage dependency of inactivation of Na^+ channels. See text for details.

channels have recovered from inactivation and returned to their original closed state so are ready to re-open in response to a depolarizing stimulus.

During the final phase of repolarization K^+ channels have generally high conductance because many K^+ currents have been activated by the depolarization, particularly I_{K1}. Until these K^+ conductances return to their resting values, a greater than normal stimulus will be required to reach the threshold for a second opening of Na^+ channels and the production of another upstroke. As the membrane potential repolarizes progressively, more Na^+ channels recover from inactivation. Therefore, a depolarizing stimulus arriving at the beginning of the relative refractory period will produce an action potential upstroke of small amplitude whilst one arriving near the end of the period will produce an upstroke of larger amplitude. The return to normal resting K^+ channel conductance marks the end of the relative refractory period.

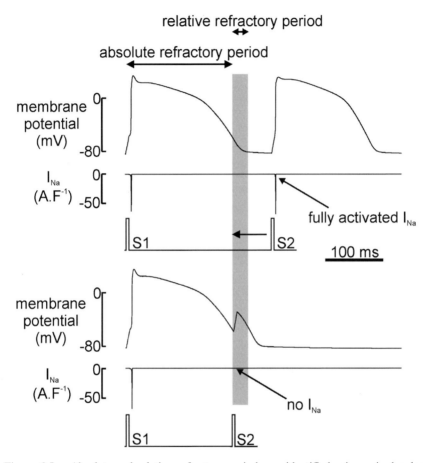

Figure 6.5.   Absolute and relative refractory periods are identified using paired pulse protocols. The first stimulus (S1) depolarizes the cells enough for I_{Na} to be activated. An action potential is produced. A second stimulus (S2) following the first produces a fully formed second action potential (upper part of figure) because I_{Na} is fully activated.   Once the interval between S1 and S2 has decreased sufficiently that no I_{Na} can be elicited by S2, no second action potential is formed (lower part of figure). The absolute refractory period has been achieved during which no propagating action potentials can be initiated no matter the stimulus strength. The small depolarization is produced by reactivation of some Ca^{2+} channels. The relative refractory period (shaded area) is the interval during which a second action potential can be elicited but the stimulus required is larger than normal.

We can see now that a rapid upstroke and fast conduction both depend on the availability of Na^+ channels. Na^+ channel inactivation is also essential for action potential repolarization because if large inward currents continue to flow until the end of the plateau the time taken for completion of phase 3 will be greatly prolonged. In this context, there are some patients with inherited forms of cardiac arrhythmia that arise from abnormalities in the Na^+ channel structure. These alter the inactivation kinetics producing larger Na^+ currents than normal during the plateau leading to early after-depolarizations, prolonged repolarization and tachyarrhythmias.

6.5.2   *Channel nomenclature*

The channel nomenclature is based on that for voltage-gated potassium and calcium channels. The name of an individual channel consists of the chemical symbol of the major permeating ion (in this case, Na^+) with the primary physiological regulator (in this case, voltage) following as a subscript (e.g. Na_V). The number after the subscript describes the gene subfamily (with Na^+ channels there is only one such subfamily discovered so far, Na_{V1}, but K^+ channels have many). The number following the decimal point identifies the channel isoform (e.g. $Na_{V1.5}$) and has been assigned roughly in the order in which the genes were identified. Splice variants of each isoform are denoted by lowercase letters following the numbers (e.g. $Na_{V1.1a}$).

6.5.3   *$Na_{V1.5}$*

The main form of cardiac Na^+ channel is known as $Na_{V1.5}$ and this gives rise to the cardiac Na^+ current. It belongs to a family with nine known members named $Na_{V1.1}$ to $Na_{V1.9}$. The names of the genes coding for these channels are SCN1A to SCN11A. Two genes – SCN6A and 7A – can, for our purposes, be ignored because they have both evolved directly from one ancestral gene and their product, called Na_x, is now known not to be voltage gated and cannot produce a rapid depolarizing current. The gene coding the main cardiac form of the channel is SCN5A. As we noted in Chapter 4, Na^+ channels comprise one so-called alpha subunit which has four (pore-forming) domains each with six trans-membrane segments. The α-subunit forms the functional channel but its kinetics and voltage dependence can be modified by its association with beta subunits.

The roles of Na^+ channel β-subunits in the heart are not well understood. We know there are four types of β-subunit each around 30–35 kDa ($Na_{V\beta1}$–$Na_{V\beta4}$). The genes coding for them have been named in the order that they were discovered: SCN1B, SCN2B, SCN3B and SCN4B. It is thought that subunits 1 and 3 interact with the α-subunit non-covalently and that subunits 2 and 4 link to the α-subunit with a disulphide bond. They do not form the ion-conducting pore but, instead, they modulate channel gating and also appear to link the channel protein to the cytoskeleton and influence its assembly with a variety of other proteins to form larger complexes. More specifically there is evidence that β-subunits are involved in Na^+ channel localization and trafficking associated with anchoring and adaptor proteins such as ankyrin and dystrophin and with caveolins.

6.5.4 *The binding of TTX*

The nine Na^+ channel isoforms have greater than 50% amino acid sequence homology in their trans-membrane and extracellular domains. $Na_{V1.1}$, $Na_{V1.2}$, $Na_{V1.3}$, and $Na_{V1.7}$ are the most closely related of the group. All four are very sensitive to TTX (with a K_d of roughly 1–10 nM) and are found widely in neurones. Their genes are all located on human chromosome 2q23-24, consistent with a common evolutionary origin. On the other hand the main cardiac isoform, $Na_{V1.5}$ (as well as the closely related channel proteins $Na_{V1.8}$ and $Na_{V1.9}$) is encoded by genes located on chromosome 3p21-24 and is much less sensitive to inhibition by TTX (with K_d values > 2 µM).

6.5.5 *The effect of local anaesthetics*

In addition to TTX, other drugs inhibit or block the channel. Most local anaesthetics fall into this category and their block of the channel underlies their use in treatments for some cardiac arrhythmias. In contrast to the action of TTX, most block from the cytoplasmic side in a voltage-dependent manner. Lidocaine, for example, is more efficacious when the cells are held at depolarized potentials, implying that the drug binds more strongly to the sodium channels when they are inactivated. It is thought that the drug stabilizes the channel in its inactivated state so preventing the transition back to a resting, closed state on repolarization of the membrane. The drug also progressively blocks more channels if they are frequently activated rather than kept in a resting unactivated (or closed) state. This drug effect is called "use-dependent block". To assess use-dependent block usually the IC_{50} (the half maximal inhibitory concentration) of the drug measured in the baseline or unstimulated condition is compared with the IC_{50} measured during stimulation or activation.

Depending on the pK of the drug molecule, at physiological pH some percentage of it will be in a charged form with the remaining percentage uncharged. (The dissociation constant (K) defines the ratio of the concentrations of the dissociated ions and the undissociated acid. The logarithm of the dissociation constant (pK) is more commonly used and is equal to $-\log_{10}K$.) Only the uncharged molecule diffuses readily across the surface membrane and, once inside the cell, this form will reach a new equilibrium with the charged species and the latter will not readily leave the cell. This charged form of the molecule binds to a site on the inside of the ion channel near its cytoplasmic face.

Sodium channel blockers are used in the treatment of some forms of cardiac arrhythmia. We will discuss these in more detail in Chapter 9. They can be classified as a Class I drug (based on the Vaughan Williams classification, which subdivided drugs on the basis of their known primary effect on the cardiac action potential at that time – 1970). Class I anti-arrhythmic agents interfere with the Na^+ channel. The rationale for their use is as follows. As we now know, the slope of the upstroke (phase 0) depends on the activation of Na^+ channels. The more channels that are activated then the faster the cell depolarizes and the faster adjacent cells will become depolarized. This leads to a more rapid transmission of action potentials between cells. Inhibition or blockade of Na^+ channels decreases the slope of the upstroke and amplitude of the action potential so reduces the speed of action potential transmission. The overall effect is a reduction in conduction velocity, which can stop abnormal re-entrant circuits that are a common cause of arrhythmia.

6.5.6 *Distribution of the Na⁺ channel*

The sub-cellular distribution of $Na_{V1.5}$ in cardiac ventricular myocytes is still being debated. A significant portion of channels are located at the intercalated discs but $Na_{V1.1}$, $Na_{V1.3}$ and $Na_{V1.6}$ have been found in addition to $Na_{V1.5}$ in the transverse tubules.   There is a heterogeneous distribution pattern of $Na_{V1.5}$ within the cardiac conduction system and across the ventricular wall that may have significant consequences in various forms of conduction abnormality and arrhythmogenesis.

To underline the importance of the channel to proper cardiac function, homozygous knock-out (KO) SCN5A mouse (SCN5A$^{-/-}$) embryos die with severe cardiac malformations whilst heterozygous KO mice (SCN5A$^{+/-}$) display slow atrial, atrioventricular and ventricular conduction and are more susceptible to ventricular arrhythmias.

6.6   Phase 1 – Early repolarization

Na^+ channel activation produces the upstroke and cells will depolarize towards E_{Na}. Na^+ channel inactivation and activation of outward currents that bring about some early repolarization often prevent the membrane potential from reaching E_{Na} and curtail the upstroke amplitude. In most cardiac myocytes there is a distinct early and partial repolarization of the membrane immediately following the upstroke and this is called phase 1. The phase is produced mainly, though not exclusively, by K^+ channels that open rapidly (within 3–10 ms) and then inactivate within about 30–40 ms (see Fig. 6.6). These channels are the major contributor to the

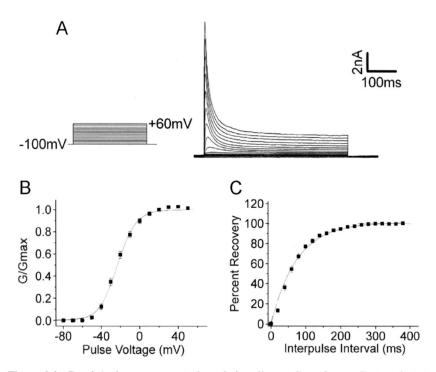

Figure 6.6. Panel A shows representative whole-cell recordings from cells transfected with human $K_{V4.2}$. A family of depolarizing clamp steps evoke progressively larger currents as the cells are clamped to more positive potentials. The current–voltage relationship from experiments like that in Panel A is illustrated in Panel B. The sizes of the currents have been scaled and expressed as a percentage of the maximum (G/Gmax). Panel C shows the results of experiments using a two-pulse clamp protocol with an increasing interpulse interval. As the interpulse interval is increased more channels recover from inactivation. Reproduced with permission from Levy *et al.* (2010) *J. Physiol.* **588**, 2657–2668.

transient outward current (I_{to}) that partially repolarizes the membrane producing the characteristic "notch" seen in recordings of action potentials.

6.6.1 *The transient outward current – I_{to}*

The transient outward current influences the balance of inward and outward currents during the plateau so it has a large influence on the duration and amplitude of phase 2. Cardiac cells express these channels to varying extents so I_{to} and therefore the size of the upstroke, the shapes and length of phase 1 and, indeed, the entire action potential duration vary depending on cell type (atrial, nodal, Purkinje or ventricular), location (atria, ventricles, base, apex, epi- or endocardium) and species. The channels have greater expression in the atria and Purkinje fibres compared with elsewhere, and in the ventricle there is more I_{to} in the epicardium compared with the endocardium.

The prominence of the notch correlates with I_{to} density. I_{to} is the major repolarizing current in adult mouse and rat atrial and ventricular cells, explaining the very short duration action potentials needed to support the fast resting heart rates (around 600 beats.min^{-1}) in these species.

6.6.1.1 $I_{to,1}$

I_{to} has two main components, one that is Ca^{2+}-independent (producing I_{to1}) and the other that shows some Ca^{2+}-dependency (creating I_{to2}). The Ca^{2+}-independent component, I_{to1}, can be further subdivided into two currents on the basis of their individual kinetics: a fast current ($I_{to1,f}$) and a slower current ($I_{to1,s}$). $I_{to1,f}$ appears to flow through channels formed by assemblies of $K_{V4.2}$ and/or $K_{V4.3}$ α-subunits encoded by the genes KCND2 and KCND3 respectively, while $I_{to1,s}$ flows through $K_{V1.4}$ channels encoded by the KCNA4 gene. $K_{V4.2}$ and $K_{V4.3}$ are members of a K^+ channel subfamily that form voltage-activated A-type K^+ channels. Current flowing through A-type channels is the predominant K^+ current in many neurons in which it plays a major role governing the discharge patterns of action potentials. Their rapid firing requires that the neurons repolarize very quickly and the rapid transient nature of the current ensures this. The subfamily of the channel group has many similarities to the Shaker K^+ channel discussed in Chapter 4 but has distinct differences in activation and inactivation kinetics, voltage sensitivity and pharmacology. They are gene products of a sister gene to the Shaker called Shal.

Whereas we have learnt so far that K^+ channels activate much more slowly than Na^+ channels and inactivate very slowly or functionally almost not at all, the A-type K^+ channels that produce $I_{to1,f}$ inactivate very rapidly. As we discussed in Chapter 4, the inactivation results from a particle (the so-called ball) that is attached to the cytoplasmic face of the channel by a protease-cleavable domain (the so-called chain), binding to a site in the conducting pathway and blocking the channel pore. Following repolarization, the inactivation particle moves away from the binding site and allows the channel to be reactivated. This mechanism is termed N-type inactivation by the "ball-and-chain" model. Whilst $I_{to,f}$ and $I_{to,s}$ activate over relatively similar time courses and voltages, they differ in two major ways. $I_{to,s}$ inactivates about two to five times more slowly than $I_{to,f}$, and all the $I_{to,f}$ is available for reactivation about 200 ms after a test step, whereas $I_{to,s}$ requires almost 10 s to evoke the maximum current (compare Fig. 6.6 Panel C with Fig. 6.7).

Another type of inactivation

The other type of inactivation, called C-type, is only now being better understood. Remember from Chapter 4 that it is the tight coordination of K^+ ions with the residues forming the selectivity filter that determines the ionic species that will pass through the pore. It appears that C-type inactivation involves subtle repositioning of residues around the selectivity filter so that its geometry changes and decreases the ability of the pore to conduct ions. The residue repositioning takes place relatively slowly compared with the N-type inactivation.

The very slow reactivation of the slow current would support the argument that it would only play a minor role in shaping phase 1 of the action potential at fast heart rates (especially in species with fast resting rates) since little current will be available at the next excitatory event.

At slower rates (particularly in the human) the differences in reactivation kinetics may be an underlying reason explaining the transmural repolarization gradients across the walls of the ventricle. Subepicardial cells recover rapidly from inactivation but sub-endocardial cells display a much slower recovery. Evidence suggests that there is a gradient of cellular expression of the $K_{V1.4}$ channel across the ventricular

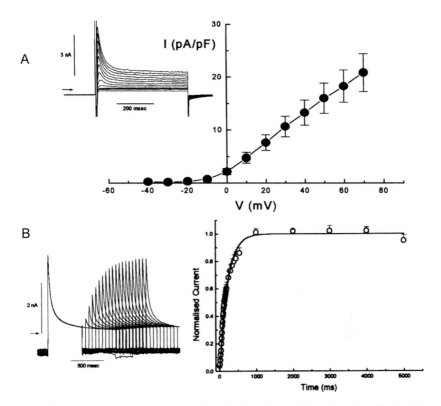

Figure 6.7. Panel A shows representative whole-cell recordings from HEK293 cells transfected with rat cardiac $K_{V4.3}$. On the left, a family of depolarizing clamp steps produces progressively larger currents as the cells are clamped to more positive potentials. The current–voltage relationship from this type of experiment is shown in the same panel on the right. Panel B shows the results of experiments using a two-pulse clamp protocol with increasing interpulse intervals. The graph on the right shows the pooled data from a number of such experiments.   As the interpulse interval is increased more channels recover from inactivation but take longer to do so compared with $K_{V4.2}$ in Fig. 6.6 Panel C. From Faivre *et al.* (1999) *Cardiovasc. Res.* **41**, 188–199 with permission.

walls so this may influence the trans-mural repolarization process. Hardly any $I_{to,f}$ flows until cells are depolarized to potentials more positive than about –35 or –40 mV. The current increases almost linearly with depolarization and typically reaches densities of about 25 A.F^{-1} with depolarizations to about +45 mV.

6.6.1.2 $K_{V4.2}$ and $K_{V4.3}$ accessory proteins

Although $K_{V4.2}$ and $K_{V4.3}$ form functional channels themselves, the binding of a β-subunit to them modulates their inactivation kinetics and rate of recovery from inactivation and may make these processes Ca^{2+} dependent. At the beginning of this section we stated that I_{to1} was generally Ca^{2+} insensitive because precisely how the β-subunits regulate $K_{V4.2/4.3}$ gating in a Ca^{2+}-dependent way remains poorly understood. There may be some Ca^{2+}-dependent inactivation of $K_{V4.3}$ but more work needs to be done to identify precise mechanisms. Association of the β-subunit with $K_{V4.2}$ and $K_{V4.3}$ also increases the peak current densities, suggesting that the subunits may also be involved in membrane expression or stabilization of the channel proteins. The beta regulatory subunits are called K^+ channel-interacting proteins (or KChIPs). There are four KChIP families but only $KChIP_2$ mRNA is abundant in heart. KChIPs bind to the N-terminal of the $K_{V4.2}$ or $K_{V4.3}$ α-subunits.   They have four EF-hand domains that bind Ca^{2+} ions so allowing $KChIP_2$ to modulate $I_{to1,f}$ in response to changes in intracellular Ca^{2+}.

EF hand proteins

The EF-hand super-family is a group of proteins that contain two alpha helices positioned roughly at right angles to each other and linked by a short loop region producing a structure somewhat similar in shape to a spread thumb and forefinger. The loop region binds Ca^{2+} ions. Mutations in the EF- hand part of the KChIP protein designed to prevent Ca^{2+} ions from binding to the loop do not alter its association with the K_v alpha subunits but disrupt KChIPs modulating effect on the K^+ channel.

6.6.1.3 I_{to2}

I_{to2} results from the activation of Ca^{2+}-sensitive chloride channels which can depolarize or repolarize cells depending on the membrane potential and E_{Cl}. At the more positive membrane potentials experienced by heart cells near the peak of their upstroke, the channels open to allow a Cl^- influx producing an outward current ($I_{Cl,Ca}$) that helps repolarize the cells towards E_{Cl}. The channels are activated by voltage but mainly by the increase in intracellular Ca^{2+} that results from its triggered release from the sarcoplasmic reticulum (SR; see Fig. 6.8). The biophysics and molecular identity of these Cl^- channels are poorly understood largely because of their scarcity in the heart. There are two likely candidates arising from two different Cl^- channel gene families: one channel type may develop from the CLCA-1 (Ca^{2+}-sensitive Cl^- channel) gene and the other from the BEST gene family. The channels are relatively non-selective compared with the more highly tuned selectivity of K^+ channels but are sensitive to changes in extracellular Cl^- concentration (Fig. 6.8B) and to known non-specific anion channel blockers. The current is sensitive to the inhibition either of Ca^{2+} release from the SR or of the L-type Ca^{2+} current (which triggers the release of Ca^{2+} from the SR). The channels are activated by cytoplasmic Ca^{2+} concentrations of between 0.2 and 5 µM. It is thought that the pool of Ca^{2+} that activates I_{to2} is Ca^{2+} released from the SR. Activation of I_{to2} hastens the speed of repolarization of phase 1. The amount of Ca^{2+} released influences the amount of repolarization and will modulate the currents activated at this point and early in phase 2.

BEST genes and bestrophin

Bestrophin proteins are encoded by the BEST genes which play a role in normal vision. Mutations in the BEST1 gene cause macular dystrophy, with one form being observed in young people where it is known as Best disease.

6.6.1.4 *Identifying components of I_{to}*

I_{to1} can be blocked by 4-aminopyridine (4-AP) but $I_{to,f}$ can be distinguished from $I_{to,s}$ and I_{to2} by using more specific inhibitors, the heteropodatoxins. These are small peptides in the venom of the giant crab spider *Heteropoda venatoria*, which alter the gating of the $K_{V4.2}$ channel or shift the voltage dependence of activation and inactivation of the $K_{V4.3}$ channel. The end result is that toxin binding either increases the probability of the channels being inactivated or changes the $V_{1/2}$ for activation so a larger depolarization is needed to open the channel. I_{to2} is not affected by 4-AP but because it is Ca^{2+} dependent, it can be altered by drugs that change cytoplasmic Ca^{2+}, e.g. caffeine, ryanodine,

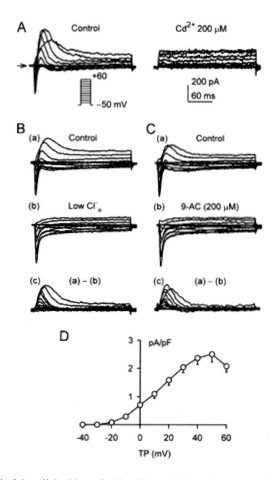

Figure 6.8. Typical I_{to2} elicited by a family of depolarizing clamp steps from −50 to +60 mV. Larger currents are produced as the cells are clamped to more positive potentials (Panel A, left) as can be seen from the current–voltage relationship in Panel D. Panel A, right shows the effect of inhibiting Ca^{2+} influx with Cd^{2+}. Panels B and C illustrate the effect on the current of decreasing the extracellular $Cl^−$ concentration and the application of 9-anthracenecarboxylic acid (9AC) respectively. From Li *et al.* (2004) *J. Mol. Cell. Cardiol.* **36**, 495–504 with permission.

nifedipine or verapamil. It is a $Cl^−$ current so it is also inhibited by anion transport blockers, e.g. SITS (4-acetamido-4'-isothiocyanostilbene-2,2'-disulphonate), DIDS (4,4'-diisothiocyano-2,2'-stilbenedisulphonic acid), 9AC (9-anthracenecarboxylic acid) or niflumic acid and, more specifically, chlorotoxin found in the venom of the scorpion, *Leiurus quinquestriatus* (see Fig. 6.8C). Inhibition of either I_{to1} or I_{to2} results in (1) the notch disappearing from recordings of the action potential and (2) a more positive early plateau. There is usually a prolongation of action potential duration but the effect of I_{to} on this is complex. A reduction in I_{to} will affect the activation, size and time course of the L-type Ca^{2+} current ($I_{Ca,L}$), because the early part of phase 1 (when this current activates) will occur over more depolarized potentials. This will result in corresponding changes in SR Ca^{2+} loading, SR Ca^{2+} release and the size of contraction.

Oligomerization domain

As mentioned earlier, voltage-gated K^+ channels are composed of four subunits, combining either as homo- or heterotetramers. Given the large number of different K^+ subunits, a considerable number of tetrameric permutations of subunits are possible. However, the combinations that emerge are limited in number because subunits from different subfamilies do not appear to form functional channels. Precisely why this occurs is not well understood, but subunits seem to be capable of recognizing favourable tetrameric combinations that are energetically stable. The area of the subunit that seems important in "recognition" is a highly conserved sequence near the cytoplasmic N terminal of the monomer, called the "T1 domain" (standing for first tetramerization domain). Mutations in the T1 domain often produce non-functional channels or simply poorly formed oligomers.

6.7 Phase 1 – Ca^{2+} influx

I_{to} is a *repolarizing* current but during phase 1 there is also a *depolarizing* current brought about by an increase in Ca^{2+} channel conductance. The current was first described in the heart (in Purkinje fibres) by Harald Reuter in a 1967 *Journal of Physiology* paper entitled: "The dependence of slow inward current in Purkinje fibres on the extracellular calcium-concentration". For a number of years there was criticism of the voltage clamp technique used because of the difficulty of ensuring good voltage control of a multicellular cardiac preparation. Although clever

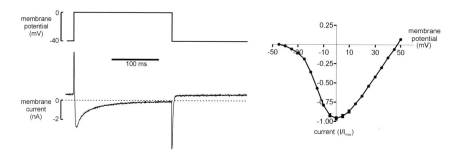

Figure 6.9. Typical $I_{Ca,L}$ recorded by holding the ventricular myocyte at −40 mV and depolarizing with a 200 ms step to 0 mV. The large excursions as the cell is clamped to 0 mV and back to −40 mV are capacitive currents. On the right is the current–voltage relationship derived from experiments like that shown on the left. The currents have been scaled and expressed as a percentage of the maximum (I/I_{max}).

modifications were implemented (e.g. three microelectrode voltage clamp) it was not until single cardiac cells could be isolated that the existence of Ca^{2+} currents could be unambiguously demonstrated. The Ca^{2+} current is much slower to activate and much smaller than the Na^{+} current and so it was originally called the "slow inward" or "second inward" current (I_{si}). It is carried by Ca^{2+} and therefore now called I_{Ca}. More specifically, it is denoted $I_{Ca,L}$ for L-type Ca^{2+} current to differentiate it from other types of currents that also have Ca^{2+} as the charge carrier (see later). The "L" stands for long-lasting, in reference to the rather slow inactivation of the current.

$I_{Ca,L}$ activates at potentials positive to −40 mV and, as Fig. 6.9 shows, its current–voltage relationship is an inverted bell-shape, reaching a maximum value around zero to +10 mV and intersecting the x-axis at about +45 mV. Note that although it is tempting to conclude that the apparent reversal potential is around +45 mV, this is not the case. E_{Ca} is about +130 mV as we calculated in Chapter 3. Direct extrapolation from the I–V relation in this case will underestimate the E_{Ca}. The reason is that free $[Ca^{2+}]$ inside the cell is about 10^{4} times smaller than the extracellular $[Ca^{2+}]$. Therefore, at potentials beyond E_{Ca} the outward driving force is not enough to produce any measurable current carried by Ca^{2+} ions although there is some electrical driving force. This means that the I–V relation tails away around +60 mV to become very small and will near the zero current level but not actually reach it until E_{Ca}. It is possible to measure an apparent E_{Ca} but this will be a reflection of the contamination of I_{Ca} records by other currents. Even if care is taken to block all other ionic channels, K^+ ions will flow in an outward direction through Ca^{2+} channels because their intracellular concentration is about 10^6 times greater than Ca^{2+}. Assuming the permeability of Ca^{2+} channels is 10^3 times larger for Ca^{2+} than K^+, it will still be possible for K^+ to be the main charge carrier through the Ca^{2+} channel at very positive potentials.

Whereas four subunits unite to form a typical K^+ channel, Ca^{2+} channels are similar in structural organization to Na^+ channels and are formed by one large protein with four homologous pore-forming domains, each containing six membrane-spanning regions. When the channel opens Ca^{2+} ions flow through it and, although the current produced does not reach a peak as quickly as I_{Na}, it nevertheless is maximal within about 2–4 ms from the start of the action potential. It is an inward current typically about 1–3 nA in a single ventricular cell.

6.7.1 *The role of $I_{Ca,L}$*

The role of the $I_{Ca,L}$ in the normal heart is to couple the electrical event (the action potential) to the production of contraction – the process known as excitation–contraction (or EC) coupling. There is an excellent book and good reviews on this topic written by Don Bers to which the reader is referred. EC coupling in the heart cannot occur in the absence of extracellular calcium as was first demonstrated by Sydney Ringer in 1883. The key step in contraction of the heart is to ensure on each excitation that Ca^{2+} is moved from the extracellular space into the cells, a transfer that produces the L-type Ca^{2+} current. Opening of the Ca^{2+} channel allows a Ca^{2+} influx through the surface membrane so the local Ca^{2+} concentration just beneath the membrane increases.

The myofibrils within the cell are surrounded by a network of interconnecting tubules and cisternae called the sarcoplasmic reticulum (SR). At multiple sites within this network, the tubule membrane

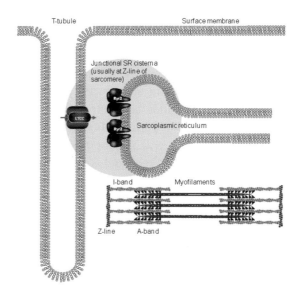

Figure 6.10.   The relationship between the junctional SR cisternae and the extensions of the surface membrane, the T-tubules. Junctional cisternae usually occur at the Z-line of the myofilaments. The "couplon" is indicated by the shaded area.

broadens to form flattened sacs, the junctional SR cisternae, which abut the surface membrane and its extensions, the transverse (T) tubules. The surface membrane and T-tubules that face the junctional SR membrane contain L-type Ca^{2+} channels. Embedded in the apposing areas of the junctional SR membrane and grouped in clusters are SR Ca^{2+} release channels, also known as "ryanodine receptors" because of their sensitivity to interference by the plant alkaloid, ryanodine. The close spatial apposition of the L-type Ca^{2+} channels and the underlying cluster of ryanodine receptors (about 6–20) at the so-called dyadic cleft is a key architectural component of the EC coupling system because both sets of channels exist in a microdomain with restricted ionic diffusion.   This local area containing the L-type Ca^{2+} channels and their adjacent ryanodine receptor clusters forms a functional Ca^{2+} release complex that has been termed a "couplon" (Fig. 6.10).

Sydney Ringer

Sydney Ringer was by all accounts an outstanding physician but his distinction lies in him being one of the first true clinician scientists. He had a busy clinical practice in central London but first thing in the morning and following his afternoon clinic he would spend time in his laboratory at University College London, where he was initially Professor of Materia Medica, then latterly Professor of Medicine and Clinical Medicine. He wrote a monograph entitled *Handbook of Therapeutics* and many papers, but it is the series in the *Journal of Physiology* in 1882 and 1883 that remain his most well known. One of these, appearing in 1883 in volume 4 pp. 29–42 entitled "A further contribution regarding the influence of different constituents of the blood on the contraction of the heart", is the most widely cited. The work detailed in this paper emphasizes that chance happenings often lie at the foundations of our understanding of biological mechanisms. Ringer was clearly a meticulous and observant scientist and openly candid about "mistakes" in his laboratory. He writes: "After the publication of a paper in the Journal of Physiology, Vol. III, No. 5, entitled – 'Concerning the influence exerted by each of the constituents of the blood on the contraction of the ventricle', I discovered, that the saline solution which I had used had not been prepared with distilled water, but with pipe water supplied by the New River Water Company. As this water contains minute traces of various inorganic substances, I at once tested the action of saline solution made with distilled water and I found I did not get the effects described in the paper referred to. It is obvious therefore that the effects I had obtained are due to some of the inorganic constituents of the pipe water." This slip up in solution preparation and its subsequently recorded effects caused Ringer to conclude: "The heart's contractility cannot be sustained by saline solution ... containing bicarbonate of soda and potassium chloride; ... a lime salt is necessary for the maintenance of muscular contractility." Ringer had the pipe water analysed and details it to have "38.3 parts per million" of calcium, which is almost 1 mM.l^{-1} Ca^{2+} (actually 0.98 mM.l^{-1}), about the levels of the ion we include in physiological salines used today. It is little wonder then that his earlier reports stated that saline comprising only Na$^+$ and K$^+$ added to the pipe water could sustain the heart function. The hard water in London ensured Ca^{2+} was already present. As well as identifying the importance of (extracellular) Ca^{2+} ions to the heart beat and its strength of contraction, Ringer established the consequence of the bathing solution and its ionic constituents to the well-being of tissues in isolation. The bathing solution or "saline" became known as "Ringer's solution" and it is still used today albeit in more modified forms. It has allowed cells and tissues to be studied *in vitro* and, just as significantly, provided the basis of intravenous saline infusions used in daily medical or surgical practice.

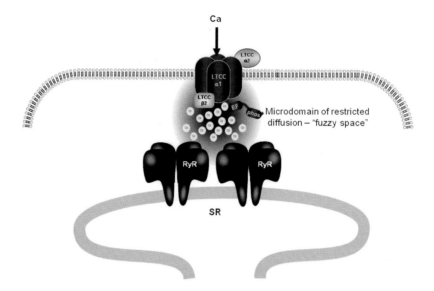

Figure 6.11. The architecture of a couplon. The close spatial apposition of the L-type Ca^{2+} channels (LTCC) and the underlying cluster of ryanodine receptors (RyR) (here just two are shown) occurs in a microdomain of restricted ionic diffusion. An L-type Ca^{2+} channel and its adjacent ryanodine receptor cluster form a functional Ca^{2+} release complex termed a "couplon". As Ca^{2+} enters the cell on opening of the L-type Ca^{2+} channels the Ca^{2+} concentration in the microdomain increases.

6.7.1.1 *SR Ca^{2+} release*

Ryanodine receptors are ligand gated with their opening dictated by the presence of Ca^{2+}. As Ca^{2+} increases in the microdomain (Fig. 6.11) more Ca^{2+} binds to the activating sites on the ryanodine receptors (two to four Ca^{2+} ions bind to each receptor) and they open. The process is known as Ca^{2+}-induced Ca^{2+} release (CICR) because the ryanodine receptors allow stored Ca^{2+} in the SR to be released into the cytoplasm producing the cytoplasmic Ca^{2+} transient that causes contraction of the myofibrils. The process is an amplification mechanism because only a small influx of Ca^{2+} into the cell is required to evoke a much larger release of Ca^{2+} from the intracellular stores. The gain of the system can be described as the total amount of Ca^{2+} released from the SR divided by the amount of Ca^{2+} influx through the L-type Ca^{2+} channel. Ca^{2+} acts as a signal transducer responding to the extracellular signalling event (the

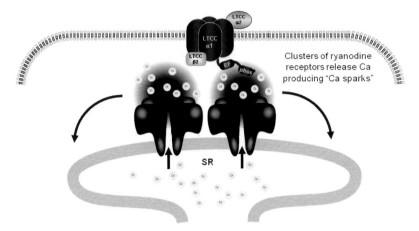

Figure 6.12. An increase in Ca^{2+} concentration in the microdomain causes the ryanodine receptors to open and release Ca^{2+} from the SR. The process is known as Ca^{2+}-induced Ca^{2+} release. The opening of a cluster of ryanodine receptors produces release events known as Ca^{2+} sparks. During the action potential the summation of thousands of these sparks produces the Ca^{2+} transient.

action potential) by activating a membrane-bound receptor (the ryanodine receptor), which in turn alters the intracellular Ca^{2+} concentration creating a contractile response. The signal transduction from L-type Ca^{2+} channel to the SR occurs within the microdomain of the dyadic cleft and produces local release events that can be observed, using imaging techniques and Ca^{2+}-sensitive fluorescent indicators, as transient increases in the concentration of intracellular Ca^{2+} confined to small (about 2–5 μm diameter) areas. Jon Lederer and colleagues coined the term "Ca^{2+} sparks" to describe these small, transient, local releases of Ca^{2+}. The "sparks" represent the building blocks of EC coupling, with the whole cell Ca^{2+} transient being produced from the temporal summation of individual Ca^{2+} sparks (Fig. 6.12).

One might expect that this EC coupling mechanism could exhibit positive feedback since Ca^{2+} released from the SR through the ryanodine receptors would itself activate neighbouring ryanodine receptors resulting in regenerative – and uncontrollable – Ca^{2+} release. The problem has been considered in great depth by Michael Stern, Mark Cannell, Ernst Niggli, Peace Cheng and a number of others.

It is now acknowledged that Ca^{2+} sparks are usually independent Ca^{2+} signalling events and do not interact with neighbouring Ca^{2+} release sites. In this way the release of Ca^{2+} and the size of the subsequent contraction is graded depending on how many L-type Ca^{2+} channels are activated. The independence of neighbouring Ca^{2+} release sites ensures stable and graded responses of the EC coupling mechanism and occurs because (1) the ryanodine receptors are relatively insensitive to activating Ca^{2+} and (2) once Ca^{2+} has left the microdomain near the release site it diffuses away rapidly so does not evoke release from its neighbouring cluster. Having more than one L-type Ca^{2+} channel per microdomain (there are maybe 10–25) creates a safety margin so that if one channel does not activate the cluster, another will.

On a beat-to-beat basis two main systems are involved in removing Ca^{2+} from the cytoplasm and so inducing relaxation. Ca^{2+} is pumped back into the SR by the sarcoplasmic/endoplasmic reticulum Ca^{2+} ATPase (SERCA2a) and extruded from the cell by the sarcolemmal Na^+/Ca^{2+} exchange (Fig. 6.13). Although cardiac cells possess other systems to decrease cytoplasmic Ca^{2+} concentration (namely the sarcolemmal Ca^{2+} ATPase and mitochondria), these contribute less than 5% towards relaxation of a normal twitch. SERCA2a and Na^+/Ca^{2+} exchange contribute about 70 and 25% respectively towards relaxation though there are species differences in the percentage contributions. In steady-state conditions the amount of Ca^{2+} leaving the cell is the same as the amount entering so that precise Ca^{2+} homeostasis is achieved.

6.7.2 *Ca^{2+} channels*

That Ca^{2+} channels exist at all was first revealed by Paul Fatt and Bernard Katz in crab muscle fibres in 1953 (remember that the separate existence of Na^+ and K^+ channels had only just been described by Hodgkin and Huxley a year earlier). After substituting Na^+ with choline in the solution bathing the fibres (akin to Hodgkin and Huxley's substitution experiments on the squid giant axon), they found that the

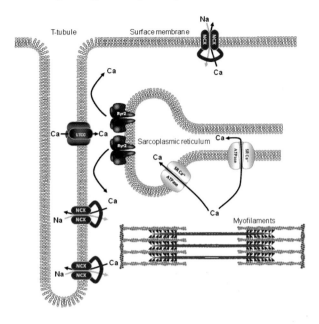

Figure 6.13.   The main systems involved in beat-to-beat cardiac cell Ca^{2+} regulation. Ca^{2+} influx through the L-type Ca^{2+} channel triggers (LTCC) the release of Ca^{2+} stored in the SR. Two main systems are involved in removing Ca^{2+} from the cytoplasm and so inducing relaxation. Ca^{2+} is pumped back into the SR by the SR Ca^{2+} ATPase and extruded from the cell by the sarcolemmal Na^+/Ca^{2+} exchange (NCX).

muscle still generated action potentials. They wrote:

> The effect of the substitution of choline for sodium was unexpected and striking; in no case were muscle fibres rendered inexcitable; on the contrary, the action potential became significantly larger, and many fibres which had previously given small local responses now produced large propagated potentials…These changes were associated with an increase in the twitch response.

There are various forms of Ca^{2+} channel and these can be classified using their electrophysiological and pharmacological properties. High voltage-activated (HVA) channels can be distinguished from low voltage-activated (LVA) channels on the basis that HVA channels only activate at membrane voltages more positive than about –30 mV. The current flowing through these channels is large and long lasting so they were called L-type channels. L-type channels can be modified by several classes of clinically useful drugs. The most widely studied of these are the dihydropyridines (e.g. nifedipine and nitrendipine), the phenylalkylamines (e.g. verapamil and D 600), and the benzothiazepines (e.g. diltiazem). In fact, the L-type Ca^{2+} channel is also known as the dihydropyridine receptor (DHPR) on account of its sensitivity to these agents. The channel can also be inhibited by some inorganic ions, e.g. Cd^{2+} and La^{3+}. LVA channels activate at more negative voltages (around −70 mV), the current carried by them activates and inactivates rapidly (i.e. is transient) and the single-channel conductance is small (tiny) so they were called T-type channels. They are insensitive to L-type channel blockers, but are inhibited by mibefradil and the inorganic ion Ni^{2+}.

A T-type Ca^{2+} channel blocker

Mibefradil was released in the United States in 1997 for the management of hypertension and chronic stable angina, but post-release surveillance indicated there were serious pharmacokinetic interactions between it and a variety of other established drug treatments for the heart, leading to its withdrawal from human use a year later. It has some L-type Ca^{2+}- and Na^+-channel blocking properties but it remains an useful pharmacological probe for investigating the contribution of, primarily, T-type Ca^{2+} channels to cardiovascular function.

A third type of channel found mainly in neurones had different behaviour from the other two in that it had a single-channel conductance of a size that lay between that of L- and T-type. This channel was called N-type (for neuronal, having neither L- nor T-type characteristics). It is now clear that there is a wide assortment of Ca^{2+} channels with a range of different behaviours presumably filling a variety of biological signalling functions. The neuronal forms of the channel could be further divided into N-, P-, Q- and R-type channels depending on their sensitivity to a variety of neurotoxins isolated from marine snails and some spiders. Finally, with the practical realization that in some cells P- and Q-type current components cannot be adequately separated, the term P/Q-type current is used. This seems appropriate because it appears that these currents arise from splice variants of the gene coding the main channel-forming (α1A) subunit. N-type channels are typically inhibited

	Type	Ca$_V$	α1 subunit	Gene	Blocker	In cardiac muscle?	Cardiac location
HVA	L	1.1	S	CACNA1S	DHP, PAA, BTZ	no, skeletal muscle	
		1.2	C	CACNA1C	DHP, PAA, BTZ, Cd^{2+}	yes	all areas
		1.3	D	CACNA1D	DHP, PAA, BTZ, Cd^{2+}	yes	SAN, atria, ventricles
		1.4	F	CACNA1F	DHP	no, retinal neurones	
	P/Q	2.1	A	CACNA1A	ω-agatoxin	no, brain, PN	
	N	2.2	B	CACNA1B	ω-conotoxin	no, brain, PN	
	R	2.3	E	CACNA1E	SNX-482, Ni^{2+}	no, brain, pancreas, kidney	
LVA	T	3.1	G	CACNA1G	mibefradil, Ni^{2+}	yes	atria, nodes
		3.2	H	CACNA1H	mibefradil, Ni^{2+}	yes	SAN
		3.3	I	CACNA1I	mibefradil, Ni^{2+}	?	SAN ?

Table 6.1.   Classification of different types of Ca^{2+} channel. DHP, dihydropyridine; PAA, phenylalkylamine; BTZ, benzothiazepine; PN, peripheral neurons; SAN, sino-atrial node. Shading denotes that the channel is expressed in the heart.

by ω-conotoxin, whereas P/Q- and R-type channels are blocked by ω-agatoxin and SNX 482 respectively.

The different subfamilies of the voltage-sensitive Ca^{2+} channels are numbered according to the L, T and N designation so that Ca$_{V1}$ are L-type channels, Ca$_{V3}$ are T-type and Ca$_{V2}$ comprise the N-, P-, Q- and R-type channels (Table 6.1). Once again, the number following the decimal point identifies the channel isoform, which has been assigned roughly in the order in which the different alpha subunits were identified. The L-type channels are named $Ca_{V1.1}$ to $Ca_{V1.4}$ and these correspond with the α1S (skeletal muscle), α1C (cardiac muscle), α1D (neuro-endocrine) and α1F subunits respectively. The T-type channels are named $Ca_{V3.1}$ to $Ca_{V3.3}$, and these relate to α1G, α1H and α1I subunits. In the Ca_{V2} subfamily, $Ca_{V2.1}$ designates channels containing the α1A subunit or P/Q-type channels, $Ca_{V2.2}$ maps to the α1B subunit and N-type channel and $Ca_{V2.3}$ is the α1E subunit and R-type channel. Despite there being many different types of Ca^{2+} channel only two exist in the heart, L- and T-type.

6.7.3 *Ca^{2+} channel structure*

By far the most common Ca^{2+} channel in the heart is the L-type channel. Like others, it is a hetero-oligomeric protein complex that can comprise up to five subunits α1, α2, β, γ and δ. The main α1-subunit (205–273 273 kDa) forms the pore and contains the selectivity filter, the voltage-sensor and the binding sites for the channel agonists and inhibitors. It shares similarities with Na^+ channel structure in that there are four homologous repeated domains (I to IV) each containing six trans-membrane segments (S1 to S6). The pore is formed by the P-loop region that links S5 and S6 of each domain (Fig. 6.14). In association with the HVA α1-subunit is the β-subunit (about 55 kDa). LVA channels do not appear to co-express with β subunits. The two subunits associate at the so-called alpha subunit interaction domain (AID), which is a highly conserved sequence of 18 amino acids between domains I and II, and the corresponding beta interaction domain (BID) located between the second and third α-helices of the β-subunit. The lone expression of the α1-subunit allows current to flow but co-expression of α1- and β-subunits increases the peak current, shifts the voltage dependence of activation and speeds the inactivation kinetics. It is thought that the β-subunit increases the number of functional channels at the membrane by improving their trafficking to the membrane and by stabilizing channel opening. There are four types of β-subunit (β1, β2, β3 and β4). The most

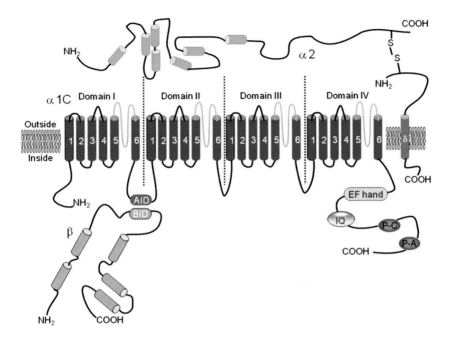

Figure 6.14.   Structure of the L-type Ca^{2+} channel.   The β-subunit associates with the α1-subunit at the alpha subunit interaction domain (AID) and beta interaction domain (BID) located on the β-subunit. The α2-subunit is located extracellularly and is linked by disulphide bonds to the δ-subunit that crosses the plasma membrane.   There are phosphorylation sites for CaM kinase (P-C) and PKA (P-A) as well as part of the protein that is important in channel inactivation situated near its carboxy terminal. The IQ domain is a conserved sequence that is involved in Ca^{2+}/CaM binding. The sub-families Ca_{V1} and Ca_{V2} have an IQ motif located near their C-termini. It is named after the isoleucine–glutamine (IQ) pair that starts the sequence (see text for more details).

dominant in the heart is β2, although β4 is highly expressed in the developing heart. Little is known about the mechanisms governing association of subunits but some preferential associations do exist – α1C with β2 in the heart for example – and such links could be regulated during development.

The α2/δ-subunits of the channels regulate peak current and the activation and inactivation kinetics.   These subunits are encoded in the same gene. The α2-subunit is located extracellularly and held by disulphide bonds to the δ-subunit that crosses the plasma membrane. The precise function of the γ-subunits is not known and although the subunit associates with the skeletal isoform of the channel, it is not certain if that is true for the cardiac forms.

6.7.3.1 *The passage of Ca^{2+} through the L-type channel*

There are two main requirements for sarcolemmal Ca^{2+} channels in the heart: firstly, they need to transport Ca^{2+} ions rapidly across the cell membrane in order to trigger the cytoplasmic Ca^{2+} transient; secondly, whilst maintaining high transport rates, they need to discriminate and selectively transfer Ca^{2+} ions from other competitors, notably the similarly sized Na^+ ions.

Na^+ ions are about 90 times more abundant than Ca^{2+} ions in the extracellular fluid so the sarcolemmal Ca^{2+} channels have evolved neatly designed selectivity mechanisms to differentiate similarly sized ionic species. To have an understanding of how Ca^{2+} ions interact with the channel we need to know about some key biophysical experiments that provided evidence of relative binding affinities. Under certain experimental conditions a variety of metal ions will pass through the Ca^{2+} channel including Ba^{2+}, Sr^{2+}, Li^+, K^+ and Na^+. Hagiwara and colleagues (in 1974) found that Co^{2+} blocked current carried either by Ba^{2+} or Ca^{2+} through the channel, but the block of the current by Co^{2+} was more effective when Ba^{2+} was the charge carrier. The blocking effect therefore depended on which ion carried current through the channel. The Ba^{2+} current was most sensitive and the Ca^{2+} current least sensitive to the action of Co^{2+}. This implies that the channel binds Ca^{2+} more tightly than Ba^{2+} since the Ca^{2+} current had the greater resistance to block. In other words, Co^{2+} could compete with Ba^{2+} for binding sites more easily than Ca^{2+}. The tighter binding is presumed to arise from parts of the pore being able to stabilize the permeant Ca^{2+} ion more effectively than one of slightly different size. However, Na^+ and Ca^{2+} ions are very similar in size so the channel has evolved two Ca^{2+} binding sites in its pore and these provide a mechanism for exclusion of Na^+.

Various experimental methods can be used to determine whether there is only one ion, or several ions, in the pore at one time. One of the most established methods is the "mole fraction" experiment in which single-channel conductance is measured with a mixture of two ions (say Ca^{2+} and Na^+) bathing the channel. The total concentration of the mixture ($[Ca^{2+}] + [Na^+]$) is fixed and the mole fraction, $[Ca^{2+}]/([Ca^{2+}] + [Na^+])$ is altered. Ca^{2+} channel current in mixtures of Ca^{2+} and Na^+ ions are smaller compared with equimolar concentrations of either ion alone. This is not what one might intuitively expect and such a finding is termed the anomalous mole fraction effect and usually interpreted as one ion partially blocking the flux of the other ion through the channel. This implies that more than one ion moves through the pore at the same time in single file so that Ca^{2+} would impede the progress of Na^+ transit and vice versa. The channel selects for Ca^{2+} over Na^+ due to the presence of high affinity binding sites for Ca^{2+} and there are two such sites in the pore. Because of these high affinity sites, under physiological conditions there will generally be one Ca^{2+} ion in the channel. If a Na^+ ion tries to enter, the electrostatic repulsion from the Ca^{2+} will force it back out again. If another Ca^{2+} enters, it has a higher affinity for the occupied site than the Na^+ ion and will destabilize the bound Ca^{2+} ion which will jump onto the next binding site and so will be "bounced" though the channel. Electrostatic repulsion provides the energy to push the Ca^{2+} ions through the pore. High affinity sites and strong repulsion are the basis for rapid transit of the ions through the pore and high selectivity.

The binding sites in question appear to be in the pore region of the channel. Each P loop supplies one glutamate residue to form a cluster of four, termed the EEEE domain. Each EEEE domain appears to be functionally split into two pairs of glutamates so that each pair carries a charge of -2 provided by their carboxylate oxygen groups, which balances the valency of each Ca^{2+} ion. The arrangement is flexible so that one pair can form an electrostatic "clasp" to grab and stabilize the ion entering the pore. The ion then can be complexed by the four glutamates to form a very high affinity site or passed onto the next pair of glutamates forming a lower affinity site if another Ca^{2+} ion approaches the pore.

6.7.3.2 *L-type Ca^{2+} channel inactivation*

Following activation the L-type Ca^{2+} current decays in spite of the maintained depolarization. Current inactivation is slower than I_{to} described earlier in this chapter and so a portion of current continues to flow inward for a substantial part of the plateau. This prolonged but gradually declining inward current flow balances the outward K$^+$ currents that start to flow later in the action potential plateau and helps prolong the duration. The process of inactivation is dependent upon both trans-membrane voltage and intracellular [Ca^{2+}] – the first termed voltage-dependent inactivation (VDI) and the second, Ca^{2+}-dependent inactivation (CDI). Early experimental evidence for the existence of both mechanisms showed that the time course of inactivation of the current is prolonged when Ba^{2+} is the charge carrier. Although slow the current still shows inactivation and without Ca^{2+} present, this is due to the VDI component. Assessing the relative contributions of CDI and VDI to the combined total inactivation of $I_{Ca,L}$ is difficult and remains uncertain mainly due to the experimental intricacy required to uniquely isolate each of the factors.

It is important for the control of the CICR process that Ca^{2+} entry through the sarcolemmal membrane is limited, otherwise premature SR Ca^{2+} re-release will occur and Ca^{2+} levels within the cell will increase. The increase could also initiate a plethora of adverse events, e.g. apoptosis, hypertrophic signalling and arrhythmias. The inactivation kinetics of $I_{Ca,L}$ will determine the duration and consequently the amount of Ca^{2+} entry during depolarization. CDI is therefore a negative feedback mechanism for regulating Ca^{2+} entry and it depends on the Ca^{2+} concentration reached in the EC coupling microdomain. Although this is determined in part by the L-type Ca^{2+} influx itself, there is general agreement that the concentration depends much more on Ca^{2+} released from the SR and, in turn, this is dependent on SR Ca^{2+} content. Because the SR Ca^{2+} content is dependent upon L-type Ca^{2+} influx, CDI therefore provides a tuned mechanism for self-limiting Ca^{2+} entry and hence regulation of Ca^{2+} levels throughout the cell. When Ca^{2+} transients are abolished (e.g. by interfering with SR Ca^{2+} release or by using high concentrations of Ca^{2+} buffer), I_{Ca} inactivation is slower.

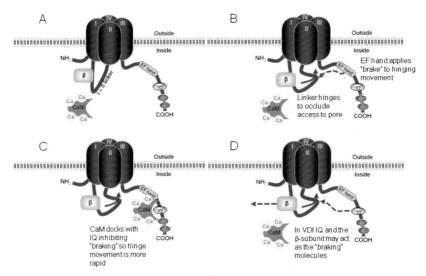

Figure 6.15. Suggested mechanism for Ca^{2+} channel inactivation. Panel A: The parts of the channel protein that are essential for CDI are located at the carboxy terminal of the α1-subunit and comprise an EF-hand Ca^{2+}-binding sequence and a series of residues that act as a calmodulin-binding site (IQ). These interact with part of the protein that links domains I and II (I–II linker) which forms part of a hinged lid blocking the pore and is important on VDI. The I–II linker has tethering sites for the β-subunit. Calmodulin (CaM) is closely associated with the Ca^{2+} channel. Panel B: CDI occurs as the I–II linker changes conformation and forms part of a hinged lid which blocks the pore. The speed of inactivation is reduced by interaction with the EF-hand part of the C-terminal tail. Panel C: As [Ca^{2+}] increases in the microdomain, Ca-CaM docks with the IQ site and this limits the restriction of the EF-hand domain and accelerates inactivation. Panel D: In VDI the I–II linker again changes conformation forming the hinged lid which blocks the pore but inactivation is slowed by interaction with the β-subunit and IQ site. Redrawn from Peterson *et al.* (2000) *Biophys. J.* **78**, 1906–1920 and Barrett & Tsien (2008) *Proc. Nat. Acad. Sci.* **105**, 2157–2162.

The parts of the channel protein that are essential for CDI are located in the proximal third of the carboxy terminal of the α1-subunit and called the Ca^{2+} inactivation, or "CI" region (Fig. 6.15). It was found that replacing the CI region by a similar region of a non-inactivating Ca^{2+} channel abolished Ca^{2+} inactivation. Conversely, substituting the CI region of the inactivating subunit into the backbone of the non-inactivating subunit conferred Ca^{2+} inactivation to the non-inactivating channel. Further experiments narrowed the parts of the protein essential for inactivation to a stretch of 53 amino acids near the beginning of the CI region that contained an EF-hand Ca^{2+}-binding sequence and a nearby region with a series of residues identified as an IQ calmodulin-binding motif (IQxxxRG). The term "IQ" refers to the first two amino acids of the motif, usually isoleucine and glutamine, and the short sequence serves as a binding site for different Ca^{2+}-binding proteins including calmodulin (CaM). Calmodulin seems to be important in Ca^{2+} inactivation because it appears to be attached to the channel almost as an integral subunit. It serves as the Ca^{2+} sensor for inactivation. As the local $[Ca^{2+}]$ increases in the microdomain, Ca^{2+} binding to CaM is favoured. The Ca^{2+}/calmodulin complex (Ca-CaM) then docks with the IQ binding motif. The resultant conformational change prevents the EF-hand domain in the CI region from interacting with the cytosolic I–II linker, which then occludes the channel pore more quickly and inactivation is accelerated (Fig. 6.15B and C).

From substitution studies we now know that the loop connecting trans-membrane domains I and II is also essential for VDI. This loop forms part of a hinged lid blocking the pore and appears to interact with the C-terminal tail. VDI involves direct obstruction of the pore by the I–II loop with the speed of inactivation in part dependent on its mobility. The mobility appears to be reduced by interaction with the membrane-anchored β2-subunit or the C-terminal tail. Thus the C-terminal tail containing the three aforementioned sites – EF hand, IQ CaM and the rest of the CI region – is thought of as a "brake" to the voltage-dependent inactivation process. When Ca^{2+} binds to CaM this brake is removed which speeds inactivation (Fig. 6.15D).

Various studies have shown that CDI is a major determinant of action potential duration. If the levels of Ca^{2+} in the cell are generally low, there will be less CDI, more L-type Ca^{2+} influx and a prolongation of inward current which will increase APD. However, VDI can also play a role in setting APD as illustrated in the effect of a G406R mutation on $Ca_{V1.2}$. This causes physiological and developmental defects associated with Timothy syndrome, a genetic disorder characterized by cardiac dysfunction and autism. The mutation greatly slows VDI, prolonging the

L-type Ca^{2+} influx and increasing APD so that arrhythmias might develop partly as a result of early afterdepolarizations (see Chapter 9).

6.7.3.3 $I_{Ca,L}$ facilitation

Changing the frequency of activation of $I_{Ca,L}$ also influences the action potential duration (APD). An increase in the frequency of current activation causes a gradual increase (or facilitation) in the peak $I_{Ca,L}$ amplitude and a slowing of inactivation of the current. It is generally agreed that facilitation requires a Ca^{2+} influx because it disappears if Ba^{2+} is used as the charge carrier or if SR Ca^{2+} release is inhibited. It has now been demonstrated by a number of groups that the effect is due to Ca^{2+}/calmodulin-dependent protein kinase II-mediated phosphorylation of the Ca^{2+} channel.   CaMK II is a serine/threonine-specific protein kinase regulated by the Ca-CaM. The catalytic site of inactive CaMK II is blocked by an auto-inhibitory part of the protein.   Unblocking of the catalytic site occurs when Ca-CaM binds to an adjacent site. The catalytic domain of CaMKII has several binding sites for ATP and the kinase transfers a phosphate group from an ATP molecule, covalently attaching it to either a serine or threonine residue with a free hydroxyl group on the target protein. The phosphorylation of, in this case, the L-type Ca^{2+} channel probably occurs at a threonine site (Thr498) on the β-subunit and this increases the open probability of the channel so $I_{Ca,L}$ increases.

6.7.3.4 Ca^{2+} channel regulation and modulation

The α1-subunit of the L-type Ca^{2+} channel also contains different phosphorylation sites for other protein kinases, such as protein kinase A and C (PKA and PKC), as well as G-protein interaction sites (Fig. 6.16). The channel function is modulated by a variety of hormones and transmitters (e.g. adrenaline and noradrenaline) that stimulate or inhibit intracellular signalling pathways via these kinases. PKA, for example, is activated by increased cyclic adenosine monophosphate (cAMP). Hormone or transmitter receptors are coupled to heterotrimeric G proteins consisting of three subunits (G_α, G_β and G_γ). When inactive, the three subunits are bound together forming a complex, $G_{\alpha\beta\gamma}$, associated at

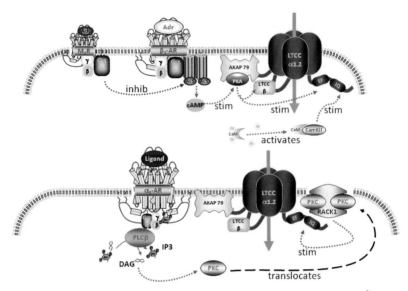

Figure 6.16.   Intracellular signalling pathways that modulate L-type Ca^{2+} channel function. Upper panel: Stimulation of the β_1 or β_2 adreno-receptor (βXAR) produces G$_{\alpha s}$-mediated activation of adenlyate cyclase (AC) and increased production of cAMP. This stimulates PKA which phosphorylates the channel at a number of sites. Muscarinic M2 receptors tend to oppose βAR stimulation of I$_{Ca}$ by acting through G$_{\alpha i}$ to inhibit AC. Lower panel: Stimulation of α_1-adrenergic, endothelin (ET), or angiotensin (AT) receptors allows G$_{\alpha q}$ to activate phospholipase C (PLC) producing diacylglycerol which, in turn, activates PKC. It is thought PKC translocates to the membrane and binds to a RACK protein (Receptor for Activated C-Kinase) near the L-type channel to be phosphorylated.

the membrane with the G$_\alpha$-subunit also bound to guanosine diphosphate (GDP). When a receptor is activated (by binding the hormone or transmitter), it catalyzes a nucleotide exchange reaction on the G$_\alpha$-subunit, GDP leaves and GTP binds which activates the G protein. The G$_\alpha$-GTP-G$_{\beta\gamma}$ complex is unstable and the G$_\alpha$-GTP and G$_{\beta\gamma}$ separate. G$_\alpha$-GTP and G$_{\beta\gamma}$ can then activate different signalling pathways and other proteins. There are many classes of G$_\alpha$-subunit but the more important in relation to cardiac function are:

(1) G$_{\alpha s}$ (also termed G$_s$ for *stimulatory*) activates adenylate cyclase stimulating the production of cAMP from ATP. cAMP acts as a second messenger in turn activating PKA.

(2) $G_{\alpha i}$ *inhibits* the production of cAMP from ATP.

(3) $G_{\alpha q/11}$ stimulates the membrane-bound enzyme phospholipase C, which in turn catalyses the formation of the second messengers, inositol trisphosphate (IP_3) and diacylglycerol (DAG) from phosphatidylinositol 4,5-bisphosphate (PtdIns(4,5)P_2 or PIP_2).

(4) $G_{\alpha 12}$ and $G_{\alpha 13}$ are used by the Rho family of signalling protein to activate some signal transduction pathways.

The sites on the channel complex that are phosphorylated have not been conclusively identified. Experimental results vary depending on how the channel complex has been reconstituted and what expression system has been used. Mutation of Ser1928 in the C-terminal portion of the α1 subunit to alanine has been found to prevent PKA phosphorylation and the consequent increase in current passed by the channel. However, it has also been demonstrated that the basal activity of $Ca_{V1.2}$ channels is decreased by mutation of Ser1700, suggesting phosphorylation of this residue might be important.

The requirement for the association of the L-type Ca^{2+} channel with A-kinase anchoring proteins (AKAPs) has also been shown. AKAPs target PKA to various substrates including the L-type channel protein. When PKA is prevented from binding to AKAPs its stimulatory effect on the channels is blocked.

Ca^{2+} channel β-subunits also have phosphorylation sites at Ser459, Ser478 and Ser479 but their precise role in bringing about an overall increase in current flowing through the channel is not well understood. In addition, there is evidence that β-adrenergic activation of $G_{\alpha s}$ can directly stimulate the L-type Ca^{2+} channel independently of PKA phosphorylation but the normal physiological role played by this pathway remains controversial. The main effect of PKA phosphorylation is an increase in P_o either as a result of changing the voltage dependence of activation or changing the gating behaviour of the channels so they are open for longer and closed for shorter periods. Phosphorylation does not result in changes to single-channel conductance or the number of channels in the membrane. For the whole cell L-type Ca^{2+} current this translates to increased peak current, quicker activation of the current and accelerated inactivation, though the latter is probably more due to enhanced CDI from the increase in peak current.

In summary, $G_{\alpha s}$-protein activation (e.g. via β-adrenoceptors) stimulates PKA, which leads to the phosphorylation of a number of key proteins involved in Ca^{2+} regulation. Phosphorylation of L-type Ca^{2+} channels results in an increase in Ca^{2+} influx. Phosphorylation of ryanodine receptors enhances SR Ca^{2+} release and phosphorylation of phospholamban results in increased activation of SERCA, which removes Ca^{2+} from the cytoplasm more rapidly hastening relaxation and increasing SR Ca^{2+} content. Phospholamban normally inhibits SERCA in its unphosphorylated state, but when the protein is phosphorylated this tonic inhibition of SERCA is removed. These (and other) intracellular events increase inotropy (the strength of contraction), lusitropy (the speed of relaxation) and chronotropy (heart rate), the latter being an effect mediated via the sino-atrial (SA) nodal cells. As L-type Ca^{2+} current increases the action potential duration would be expected to increase because there is more depolarizing current maintaining the plateau at more positive potentials. However, other mechanisms will be affected by the increase in Ca^{2+} influx (e.g. the VDI mechanism of $I_{Ca,L}$ and activation of Ca^{2+}-dependent I_{to2}) which tend to repolarize the cells more quickly. The final effect on the action potential duration will be the result of combining the different responses of the ion channels. $G_{\alpha i}$-protein activation (e.g. via adenosine or muscarinic receptor activation) reduces PKA activation and so decreases both Ca^{2+} influx and SR Ca^{2+} release. PKC regulation of L-type Ca^{2+} channels remains understudied. There is contradictory evidence that activation of PKC can stimulate or inhibit the channels. It may be that different PKC isoforms have different effects depending on how they are activated.

6.7.4   *T-type Ca^{2+}channels in the heart*

T-type Ca^{2+} current densities are highest in the pacemaker and conducting cells and are either greatly reduced or non-existent in ventricular myocytes. The current densities in the heart are highest around birth then gradually decrease but may reappear in some conditions such as cardiac hypertrophy, which appears to trigger a return to the neonatal pattern of gene expression, leading to a re-expression of T-type current particularly in ventricular myocytes. The voltage threshold for their activation is about -50 mV reaching a peak around -30 mV with a $V_{1/2}$ of about -40 mV. The current passing through them is small, about 100–200 pA. Since they do not contribute to the ventricular action potential but play a large role in shaping the action potential in pacemaker tissue, we will not discuss them further at present but will do so in more detail in Chapter 9.

6.8 Summary

- The ventricular action potential has a long duration compared with nerve. The duration of the ventricular action potential controls the duration of contraction of the cells and a long, slow contraction is required to produce an effective pump. The long action potential also produces a long refractory period which prevents the heart from contracting prematurely or contractions fusing. A typical ventricular action potential can be split into five phases.
- Phase 0 is the rapid upstroke carried by Na^+ current flowing through $Na_{V1.5}$ channels. The channels are activated by small depolarizations of neighbouring cells sensed by the S4 and "voltage-sensor paddle" regions of the Na^+ channels. At voltages more negative than -75 mV few channels activate, but as membrane potential becomes more positive more channels open with the relation steepest between -50 and -25 mV.
- Na^+ channels inactivate even though the cells remain depolarized. Inactivation involves a loop of peptide linking the S3 and S4 domains that reacts to depolarization more slowly than the initial protein movements occurring on channel opening. It hinges to block the channel conduction pathway. Inactivated Na^+ channels cannot be reactivated directly to their conducting state but must be removed by repolarization.
- While Na^+ channels are inactivated no action potential can be initiated, regardless of the stimulus strength accounting for the

absolute refractory period (in whole heart preparations called the effective refractory period). Once the membrane repolarizes to a point where a portion of Na^+ channels recover from inactivation and return to their original closed state they can re-open in response to a depolarizing stimulus. This is the relative refractory period when an action potential can be elicited but the stimulus required is larger than normal.

- In ventricular myocytes there is a distinct early and partial repolarization of the membrane immediately following the upstroke called phase 1. The phase is produced mainly, though not exclusively, by K^+ channels that open rapidly (within 3–10 ms) and then inactivate within about 30–40 ms and contribute to the transient outward current (I_{to}).

- I_{to} has two main components, one mainly Ca^{2+} independent (I_{to1}) and the other that shows some Ca^{2+} dependency (I_{to2}). I_{to1} can be further subdivided into two currents on a kinetic basis: fast current ($I_{to1,f}$) and a slower current ($I_{to1,s}$). $I_{to1,f}$ flows through assemblies of $K_{V4.2}$ and/or $K_{V4.3}$ subunits, while $I_{to1,s}$ flows through $K_{V1.4}$ channels. I_{to2} carried by Ca^{2+}-sensitive chloride channels that open to allow a Cl^- influx producing an outward current ($I_{Cl,Ca}$) that helps repolarize the cells towards E_{Cl}. These channels are activated mainly by the increase in intracellular Ca^{2+} that results from its triggered release from the SR.

- Ca^{2+} influx also occurs during phase 1 via an L-type Ca^{2+} current ($I_{Ca,L}$) that activates at potentials positive to -40 mV and reaches a maximum value at $+10$ mV. This current inactivates slowly. Its main role is to couple the electrical event (the action potential) to the production of contraction – the process known as excitation–contraction (or EC) coupling. Ca^{2+} influx through the surface membrane promotes further release of stored Ca^{2+} from the SR via the SR Ca^{2+}-release channel (the ryanodine receptor) by a process known as Ca^{2+}-induced Ca^{2+} release. Two main systems are involved in removing Ca^{2+} from the cytoplasm and so inducing relaxation. Ca^{2+} is pumped back into the SR by a Ca^{2+}ATPase (SERCA) and extruded from the cell by the sarcolemmal Na^+/Ca^{2+} exchange. The phasic increase and decrease of Ca^{2+} that gives rise to the elements of contraction and relaxation respectively is generally termed the "Ca^{2+} transient". "Ca^{2+} sparks" describe small, transient, local releases of Ca^{2+} from a cluster of ryanodine receptors. The whole cell Ca^{2+} transient is produced from the temporal summation of individual Ca^{2+} sparks.

- L-type Ca^{2+} channels are hetero-oligomeric protein complexes that can comprise up to five subunits α_1, α_2, β, γ and δ. There are different subfamilies of voltage-sensitive Ca^{2+} channels. Ca^{2+} ions move through their channels by a "Newton's cradle" mechanism whereby an ion entering the pore causes, by electrostatic repulsion, the ion in the pore to jump onto the next binding site and it "bounces" though the channel. The process of Ca^{2+} channel inactivation is dependent upon both trans-membrane voltage and intracellular $[Ca^{2+}]$ – the first termed voltage-dependent inactivation (VDI) and the second, Ca^{2+}-dependent inactivation (CDI).

- Ca^{2+} channels can undergo gradual increases in the peak $I_{Ca,L}$ amplitude accompanied by a slowing of inactivation of the current (facilitation). Facilitation is due to Ca^{2+}/calmodulin-dependent protein kinase II-mediated phosphorylation of the Ca^{2+} channel. Ca^{2+} channels can also be phosphorylated by the classical G-protein cascade. $G_{\alpha s}$-protein activation (via β-adrenoceptors) stimulates PKA, which leads to the phosphorylation of the channels resulting in increased Ca^{2+} influx.

6.9 Questions

(1) Outline the differences in EC coupling between skeletal and cardiac muscle.

(2) What is the function of T-tubules?

(3)   Calculate E_{Na} given normal intracellular and extracellular $[Na^+]$ of 10 and 140 mM respectively. Why might this value not be reached in recordings of the upstroke of the action potential?

(4) I_{to} shows inactivation. How does this occur?

(5)   What mechanisms underlie the inactivation of the L-type Ca^{2+} current?

6.10 Bibliography

6.10.1 *Books and reviews*

Bers, D.M. (2001). *Excitation–Contraction Coupling and Cardiac Contractile Force* (2nd edn). Kluwer Academic.

Bers, D.M. (2002). Cardiac excitation–contraction coupling. *Nature* **415**, 198–205.

Catterall, W.A. (2000). Structure and regulation of voltage-gated Ca^{2+} channels. *Ann. Rev. Cell. Dev. Biol.* **16**, 521–555.

Catterall, W.A. (2000). From ionic currents to molecular review mechanisms: the structure and function of voltage-gated sodium channels. *Neuron* **26**, 13–25.

Kamp, T.J. and Hell, J.W. (2000). Regulation of cardiac L-type calcium channels by protein kinase A and protein kinase C. *Circ. Res.* **87**, 1095–1102.

Sheets, M.F., Fozzard, H.A., Lipkind, G.M. and Hanck, D.A. (2010). Sodium channel: molecular conformations and antiarrhythmic drug affinity. *Trends Cardiovasc. Med.* **20**, 16–21.

6.10.2 *Original papers*

Barrett, C.F. and Tsien, R.W. (2008). The Timothy syndrome mutation differentially affects voltage- and calcium-dependent inactivation of CaV1.2 L-type calcium channels. *Proc. Nat. Acad. Sci.* **105**, 2157–2162.

Cheng, H., Lederer, W.J. and Cannell, M.B. (1993). Calcium sparks: elementary events underlying excitation-contraction coupling in heart muscle. *Science* **262**, 740⁻744.

Faivre, J.-F., Calmels, T.P.G., Rouanet, S. *et al.* (1999). Characterisation of Kv4.3 in HEK293 cells: comparison with the rat ventricular transient outward potassium current. *Cardiovasc. Res.* **41**, 188–199.

Fatt, P. and Katz, B. (1953). The electrical properties of crustacean muscle fibres. *J. Physiol.* **120**, 171–204.

Hagiwara, S., Fukuda, J. and Eaton, D.C. (1974). Membrane currents carried by Ca, Sr, and Ba in barnacle muscle fiber during voltage clamp. *J. Gen. Physiol.* **63**, 564–578.

de Leon, M., Wang, Y., Jones, L. *et al.* (1995). Essential Ca^{2+}-binding motif for Ca^{2+}-sensitive inactivation of L-type Ca^{2+} channels. *Science* **270**, 1502–1506.

Levy, D.I., Cepaitis, E., Wanderling, S. *et al.* (2010). The membrane protein MiRP3 regulates Kv4.2 channels in a KChIP-dependent manner. *J. Physiol.* **588**, 2657–2668.

Li, G.-R., Sun, H., To, J. *et al.* (2004). Demonstration of calcium-activated transient outward chloride current and delayed rectifier potassium currents in swine atrial myocytes. *J. Mol. Cell. Cardiol.* **36**, 495–500.

López-López, J.R., Shacklock, P.S., Balke, C.W. and Wier, W.G. (1995). Local calcium transients triggered by single L-type calcium channel currents in cardiac cells. *Science* **268**, 1042⁻1045.

Makielski, J.C., Sheets, M.F., Hanck, D.A. *et al.* (1987). Sodium current in voltage clamped internally perfused canine cardiac Purkinje fibres. *Biophys. J.* **52**, 1–11.

Peterson, B.Z., Lee, J.S., Mulle, J.G. *et al.* (2000). Critical determinants of Ca^{2+}-dependent inactivation within an EF-hand motif of L-type Ca^{2+} channels. *Biophys. J.* **78**, 1906–1920.

Reuter, H. (1967). The dependence of slow inward current in Purkinje fibres on the extracellular calcium-concentration. *J. Physiol.* **192**, 479–792.

Ringer, S. (1883). A further contribution regarding the influence of different constituents of the blood on the contraction of the heart. *J. Physiol.* **4**, 29–42.

Sakakibara, Y., Furukawa, T., Singer D.H. *et al.* (1993). Sodium current in isolated human ventricular myocytes. *Am. J. Physiol.* **265**, H1301–H1309.

Shacklock, P.S., Wier, W.G. and Balke, C.W. (1995). Local Ca^{2+} transients (Ca^{2+} sparks) originate at transverse tubules in rat heart cells. *J. Physiol.* **487**, 601–608.

Stern, M.D. and Lakatta, E.G. (1992). Excitation-contraction coupling in the heart: the state of the question. *FASEB J.* **6**, 3092–3100.

Chapter 7

Currents Flowing During the Later Part of the Ventricular Action Potential

In this chapter we will describe the currents that flow during the later parts of the ventricular action potential. Unlike the last chapter, in which the currents were described as far as possible in the chronological order of their occurrence, a sequential description will not be followed precisely. The reason for this is that the currents involved in repolarization overlap much more in time than currents flowing earlier in the action potential. After the very early excitatory events of phases 0 and 1, the ventricular cells remain depolarized, the trans-membrane voltage remains relatively stable so the action potential becomes quite flat as it enters the plateau or phase 2. The main features of this phase are that initially the membrane potential does not change very much but latterly it gradually becomes more negative as the cells begin to repolarize.

7.1 Chapter objectives

After reading this chapter you should be able to:
- Understand the concept of inward rectification and explain why it underlies the long cardiac action potential
- Describe the roles of the delayed rectifier currents in the repolarization process
- Explain other ion movements that occur later in the ventricular action potential

7.2   Phase 2

The maintenance of the plateau and the very slow change in membrane potential arise because the inward depolarizing currents very closely balance the outward repolarizing ones. The outward currents that now start to activate do so relatively slowly so they do not "overwhelm" the inward currents. Antagonism is minimized so that there is economy of current flow. This economy is due in large part to ventricular myocytes possessing a type of K^+-selective channel called the inward rectifying K^+ channel through which I_{K1} flows. This K^+ channel has peculiar characteristics that limit its size at depolarized potentials so that a large outward K^+ current does not occur and the action potential remains prolonged. In fact, total membrane conductance is lower during phase 2 than during phase 4. It is appropriate at this point to discuss this current in more detail, not because it flows at this point in the action potential – it doesn't – but because its unusual voltage dependence plays an important role in supporting phase 2 and shaping the ventricular action potential.

In 1949 Silvio Weidmann arguably made the first accurate recording of the cardiac action potential from the heart of a dog. A few years later Weidman demonstrated that heart cells depolarized when the extracellular $[K^+]$ was decreased, a result that initially puzzled many researchers because the cells ought to have hyperpolarized under those conditions. Weidmann's demonstration was the first illustration of the presence of a current now known as I_{K1} (and its behaviour can now be explained by the effect of extracellular $[K^+]$ on ion flow through the channels).

7.2.1 I_{K1}

To be able to discuss the basic properties of the channels through which I_{K1} flows we need to define the term "inward rectification". In Chapter 2 we showed that in an equivalent electrical circuit, ion channels could be thought of as variable resistors with the current flowing through them driven by the electrochemical gradient (the batteries). The resistors would have a linear current–voltage (I–V) relationship (i.e. one that follows Ohm's law $V = IR$; see Chapter 3, p. 37). In contrast, rectification is said to occur when the *I–V* relationship is not linear so that the conductance of a channel is not constant but varies with voltage. In other words, if a channel preferentially allows more current to flow in one direction than the other, the channel is a rectifier.

The electrical analogy is that of the function of a diode. When the diode is forward biased so that a positive voltage is applied to its anode with respect to the cathode, its effective resistance is very low (like a closed switch) so current can flow from the anode to the cathode easily. However, when the diode is reverse biased so that the voltage applied to the anode is negative with respect to the cathode, the effective resistance is very high (like an open switch) and no current flows (Fig. 7.1A). In the heart, the channel carrying I_{K1} passes inwardly directed current at potentials more negative than E_K but it passes progressively less current in the outward direction as more positive potentials are reached producing a characteristic "n-shape" *I–V* relationship. At membrane potentials more positive than about –60 mV fewer channels are activated and at about –20 mV all channels are closed. This behaviour is typical of inwardly rectifying K^+ channels (Fig. 7.1B) (see also Sakmann and Trube (1984)). However, activation of I_{K1} does not depend on membrane potential alone but also on the extracellular $[K^+]$.   Notice that if extracellular $[K^+]$ is increased there is a rightward shift in the *I–V* relationship leading to a "crossover" of outward currents because the maximum values of these are larger at increased extracellular $[K^+]$ and this leads to a shorter APD (Fig. 7.1B). This suggests K^+ ions passing through the channel or bound to the extracellular part of the channel modify the channel gating in some way.

At negative membrane potentials I_{K1} is much larger than any other repolarizing current and so it clamps the resting membrane potential close to E_K. The *I–V* relationship of I_{K1} at E_K is relatively steep indicating a low membrane resistance. The low membrane resistance means that a large amount of current needs to flow to change the membrane potential significantly so that the membrane potential is well clamped and stable until the arrival of a larger depolarizing, excitatory event. Following phase 0 the inward rectifying channels close immediately and remain

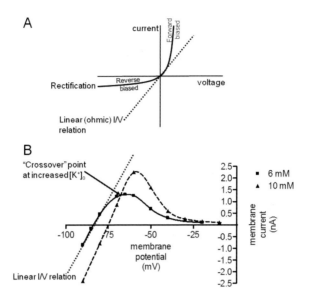

Figure 7.1. Panel A: The *I–V* relationship of a diode. When forward biased (a positive voltage applied to the anode) large currents flow from the anode to the cathode easily. When reverse biased (a negative voltage applied to the anode with respect to the cathode) negligible current flows. The dotted line indicates a *I–V* relationship that follows Ohm's law. Panel B: In an analogous way, there is a large amount of inward current in channels carrying I_{K1} at potentials more negative than E_K but less current as more positive potentials are reached. At membrane potentials more positive than about – 60 mV fewer channels are activated and at about –20 mV all channels are closed. The channels can be described as behaving like rectifiers. Increasing extracellular [K$^+$] from 6 mM to 10 mM causes a shift in the relation to the right and an increase in the maximum current.

closed for much of the plateau. The almost zero I_{K1} at the early plateau potentials prevents a rapid termination of the action potential and a loss of K$^+$ from the cells. As repolarization proceeds the inward rectifying channels tend to open again at potentials negative to –20 mV and contribute to terminating the plateau and producing phase 3 of repolarization. I_{K1} stabilizes the resting membrane potential and determines the cell input resistance, that is, the resistance of the membrane at rest.

I_{K1} density is higher in ventricular than in atrial myocytes though similar in density across the ventricular wall. Its density is very low in sino-atrial and atrio-ventricular nodal cells so their maximum diastolic membrane potentials are more depolarized than atrial and ventricular myocytes and not clamped near E_K.

7.2.1.1 *The mechanisms underlying inward rectification*

The main mechanism producing the inward rectifiying behaviour is a voltage-dependent block of the channel pore by endogenous intracellular cations. Once the channel is open, intracellular Mg^{2+} enters and blocks the pore by binding to a glutamic acid residue on the second trans-membrane domain. The concentration of Mg^{2+} at which half the binding sites are occupied is about 10 µM (at +30 mV) so at physiologically relevant concentrations of cytoplasmic Mg^{2+} (usually about 1 mM), the block of the channel occurs extremely quickly. Site-directed mutagenesis studies suggest the blocking – and hence the rectification – depends on negatively charged glutamic (D172) and aspartic acid (E224 and E299) residues located in the second trans-membrane domain and the carboxy terminal of the protein. Removing the charge on the amino acids reduces the Mg^{2+} block.

However, rectification of these channels is still observed in the absence of Mg^{2+} and it was discovered that intracellular polyamines also block them. The greater charge on the polyamine, the more potent the block of the channels. The tetravalent spermine and trivalent spermidine have more potent blocking action compared with the divalent putrescine and with Mg^{2+}. The polyamines are thought to bind to similar sites on the protein as Mg^{2+} (Fig. 7.2). Polyamines are present in almost all cells. Putrescine and cadaverine are synthesized by decarboxylation of ornithine and lysine respectively, while spermidine and spermine are synthesized from putrescine and decarboxylated S-adenosylmethionine. The polyamines or Mg^{2+} unplug from the channel at negative voltages and so the channel can conduct again.

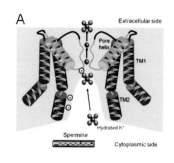

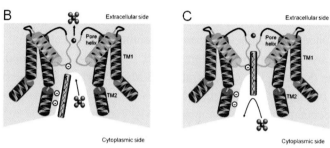

Figure 7.2. A proposed mechanism for block of the inward rectifying channel carrying I_{K1}. Panel A shows K^+ ions moving through the channel. Panels B and C: Spermine (and other polyamines) is thought to bind to similar sites on the protein as Mg^{2+}, namely in the cytoplasmic vestibule and near the selectivity filter. By doing so they impede the movement of K^+ ions through the channel.

7.2.1.2 *Structure of K_{ir} channels*

Whereas K_V channels form as an assembly of four α-subunit proteins each consisting of six membrane-spanning α-helical segments, S1 to S6, K_{ir} channels are built from four subunits each composed of just two membrane-spanning α-helices (called M1 and M2) with a type of P loop (called the H5 region) joining the two together. The channels are generally homo-tetrameric co-assemblies but some are heteromeric in structure. The voltage sensor or S4 segment is not present and, as a result, K_{ir} channels are insensitive to membrane voltage. As we just described, their opening and closing are dictated by polyvalent cation blocking and unblocking which are, however, voltage-dependent processes.

There are seven subfamilies of K_{ir} channels, denoted K_{ir1}–K_{ir7}, and each subfamily has a variable number of isoforms and degrees of rectification. The subfamilies can be divided into four groups loosely based on their functional characteristics:

(1) Strongly rectifying "classical" K_{ir} channels ($K_{ir2.x}$)
(2) G-protein gated K_{ir} channels ($K_{ir3.x}$)
(3) ATP-sensitive K^+ channels ($K_{ir6.x}$)
(4) K^+-transport channels ($K_{ir1.x}$, $K_{ir4.x}$, $K_{ir5.x}$, and $K_{ir7.x}$)

Channels through which cardiac I_{K1} flows are probably formed from $K_{ir2.1}$ and $K_{ir2.2}$ subunits coded by the genes KCNJ2 and KCNJ12 respectively.

7.2.1.3 *The effects of hypo- and hyperkalaemia on I_{K1}*

The modulation of I_{K1} by $[K^+]_o$ has important pathophysiological and clinical implications. $[K^+]_o$ can change locally in the heart in a variety of circumstances. This is because K^+ ions can accumulate in T-tubules. The T-tubule network has a mean diameter of about 200 nm which restricts ion diffusion. The diffusion rate for K^+ in the T-tubules is about nine times slower than in free solution so, following increases in heart rate or a period of ischaemia, K^+ ions accumulate in the confined spaces, producing cell depolarization because E_K becomes more positive. The depolarization causes inactivation of a portion of Na^+ channels so fewer Na^+ channels are available for activation and therefore less current is generated to form the upstroke of the action potential. The result is that phase 0 is smaller in size and the voltage change less rapid. I_{K1} channels are localized in the T-tubules so are modulated by the local changes in $[K^+]_o$ more so than if they were predominantly on the surface of the cell. The increase in $[K^+]_o$ increases the conductance of I_{K1}. Under this condition more Na^+ influx will be required to overcome the stronger repolarizing effect of the increased outward K^+ flux and so this further limits the size of the depolarizing upstroke and reduces its speed.

7.3 Phase 2 continued

The plateau is maintained by the inward depolarizing currents gradually reducing in size because their respective channels are becoming more inactivated and the outward repolarizing currents starting to slowly activate so increasing in size and opposing the former. There is a complex interplay between current flows. There are three main K^+ currents that now start to flow – I_{Kur}, I_{Kr}, and I_{Ks}, standing for ultra-rapid, rapid and slow respectively. It is important to realize that these currents do not flow in all cells of the heart. Their presence depends on species and heart tissue type (i.e. chamber or node). For example, I_{Kr} is essentially responsible for plateau repolarization in rat ventricle while I_{Ks} seems to be the dominant current for the process in guinea-pig ventricular cells. I_{Kur} seems to be largely confined to atrial cells.

7.3.1 I_{Kur}

Of the three K^+ currents, I_{Kur} is the most difficult to consistently isolate and identify. This has resulted in the current being known by a variety of names as various investigators used different terms for what, with hindsight, is probably the same current. I_{Kur} is an outwardly rectifying current that rapidly activates when the membrane potential is in the range 0 to +60 mV within about 10 ms of the voltage change, and thereafter partially inactivates over about 250 ms. Most early experiments on the current were done at room temperature and this not only slows the activation kinetics, but also greatly hinders the inactivation process such that current flow is maintained for long periods (seconds). As a result, the current was termed steady-state (I_{ss}) or sustained (I_{sus}) or sustained outward current (I_{so}). These terms become quite confusing when considering the current at normal physiological temperature because it undergoes much more rapid inactivation and so it is better to use the term ultra-rapid potassium current – I_{Kur}. The mechanism of inactivation of the channel appears akin to N-type inactivation (see Chapter 6, p. 146).

The channel through which this current flows is $K_{V1.5}$, which is encoded by the gene KCNA5. Both the mRNA and the expressed protein are found in the atria and ventricles of many species but the current is generally absent in ventricular myocytes, suggesting its appearance relies on the presence of modulating subunits or important scaffolding or trafficking proteins. The $K_{V1.5}$ α-subunit consists of the typical voltage-sensitive K^+ channel template of a tetramer of six trans-membrane segments with a P loop between S5 and S6. $K_{V\beta}$ subunits bind to control channel trafficking and also appear to influence the activation and inactivation of the channel by moving the $V_{\frac{1}{2}}$ to more negative potentials. There is also some evidence that KChIP2 (see Chapter 6, p. 148) modifies the activation and inactivation properties. The current is difficult to separate from I_{to} but the main strategy involves the use of the different sensitivities of the currents to 4-aminopyridine (4-AP). Like I_{to}, the $K_{V1.5}$ current can be inhibited by 4-AP ($K_d \approx 270$ μM) but is much more sensitive to block by the drug than the former ($K_d \approx 5.2$ mM). Following a voltage clamp step to +50 mV a brief outward current that persists in 1–5 mM 4-AP can be elicited followed by a longer lasting outward current which is sensitive to 0.25–0.5 mM 4-AP (Fig. 7.3). The rapid and brief current is I_{to} and the longer lasting current I_{Kur}. Another strategy involves using lower temperature to slow the inactivation of both currents. In Fig. 7.3A a series of 1 s test steps produces I_{to} and the current flowing at the end of the steps is due either to a portion of I_{to} that has not yet inactivated or to I_{Kur}. At 25 °C I_{to} recovers from inactivation very slowly, so if the first clamp steps are followed by a brief return to the holding potential then a second series of test pulses, I_{Kur} can be studied cleanly because I_{to} is inactivated due to the pre-pulse. At 25 °C inactivation of I_{Kur} is also slow so the current is observed (Fig. 7.3A right panel) to be rapidly activating with very little inactivating component.

At physiological temperature (Fig. 7.3C), the pre-pulse inactivation strategy for I_{to} does not work because the current recovers from inactivation much more quickly so that the short time of clamp at the holding potential (here 25 ms) allows a proportion of channels carrying I_{to} to recover from inactivation. Applying another series of test steps thereafter elicits substantial I_{to} again.

It is likely that in atrial myocytes rapid activation of I_{Kur} occurs during the latter part of phase 1 and the early part of phase 2 at a similar time as the large depolarizing $I_{Ca,L}$. This would offset the depolarization

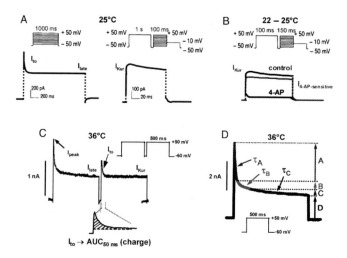

Figure 7.3. Different methods to separate I_{to} from I_{Kur} (in human atrial myocytes from non-fibrillating atria). Panel A: I_{to} and I_{Kur} at 25 °C. Currents during a 1 s long test pulse (left tracing) and during a 100 ms long test pulse (right tracing). The right tracing was preceded by a 1 s prepulse to +50 mV 20 ms before the test pulse, but for clarity only the current flowing during a test step to +50 mV is shown. I_{to} and I_{Kur} as indicated. Panel B: the effect of 1 mM 4-AP on I_{Kur} and 4-AP-sensitive current, i.e. I_{Kur} (red). Similar protocol as in Panel A but shorter pre-pulse. Panel C: I_{to} and I_{Kur} recorded at 36 °C. Current tracing during two 500 ms long test steps to +50 mV, separated by 25 ms at the holding potential of −60 mV. I_{to} recovers rapidly at this temperature and can be estimated by the area under the curve during the first 50 ms (AUC_{50ms}) of the second test pulse. Panel D: I_{to} and I_{Kur} in response to a 500 ms test pulse from −60 to +50 mV at 36 °C. A tri-exponential curve was fitted to the current trace, where τ_A is the time constant of inactivation for I_{to} and τ_B and τ_C are time constants for fast and slow inactivation, respectively, of I_{Kur}. From Ravens and Wettwer (2011) *Cardiovasc. Res.* **89**, 776–785 with permission.

produced by the Ca^{2+} influx leading to a more negative plateau potential that is observed in atrial cells, compared with ventricular myocytes where the current is essentially absent.

$K_{V1.5}$ channels could be promising drug targets for the treatment of atrial fibrillation. Atrial fibrillation (AF) is the most common sustained heart rhythm disturbance taking the form of an irregular and often abnormally fast heart rate. Whilst not generally life threatening, it can lead to unpleasant symptoms such as palpitations and shortness of breath as well as more serious complications such as stroke.

Pharmacological interventions that inhibit specific K^+ currents can be complicated to design (as we will see later in this chapter) but because I_{Kur} is largely absent in the ventricle, drugs specifically targeting the current may provide a selective therapy for AF. Inhibition of I_{Kur} would prolong the atrial action potential thereby increasing the effective refractory period and reducing the chances of re-excitation. Less obviously, block of the current would lead to a more positive early plateau potential in a range where more $I_{Ca,L}$ might be activated. This would increase Ca^{2+} influx and lead to an increase in atrial contraction. AF can cause a decrease in atrial contraction and current drugs used for rhythm control (propafenone, flecainide, sotalol, dofetilide and amiodarone) all tend to have a negative inotropic effect. Therefore, alterations to I_{Kur} may provide a way of reducing fibrillation and increasing atrial contraction.

7.3.2 I_{Kr}

Channels that carry I_{Kr} are activated at potentials more positive than -40 mV, i.e. during the plateau phase (phase 2). The $V_{1/2}$ (voltage required for half activation) is about -30 mV. However, the behaviour of the channel is not typical of a delayed rectifier (see Chapter 3, p. 46) because at voltages positive to about 0 mV, the channel very rapidly inactivates reducing outward current at this and more positive potentials. In fact, simply in terms of the I–V relation, the channel behaves like an inward rectifier shutting off at more positive voltages. The reason for this apparent behaviour is that channel inactivation develops faster than channel activation at positive potentials and so limits the amount of time that these channels spend in an open state. As the action potential moves into late phase 2 and early phase 3 and the membrane potential becomes more negative than 0mV, the channels recover from inactivation and open again. This leads to further outward current that helps with early phase 3 repolarization. The current then decreases near the end of theaction potential because of channel deactivation. This activity results

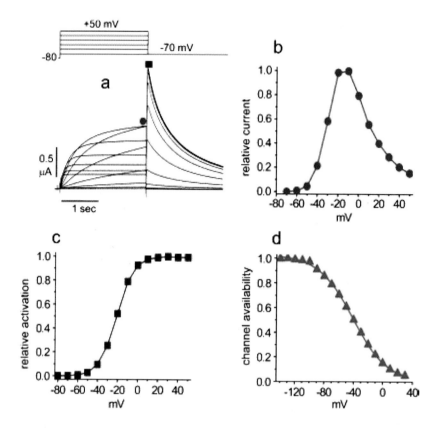

Figure 7.4. Recordings and properties typical of I_{Kr}. Panel A: the voltage clamp protocol is shown in the upper panel and evoked currents from heterologously expressed hERG channels in a *Xenopus* oocyte are shown in the lower panel. Test potentials ranged from −70 to +50 mV and deactivating "tail" currents were measured at −70 mV. Panel B: The *I–V* relationship measured at the end of the test pulses (at red circle in Panel A). Panel C: Voltage dependence of hERG activation. The peak of the tail currents measured at −70 mV (blue square in Panel A) were calculated as a percentage of the largest current and plotted as a function of the test potential. Panel D: Voltage dependence of hERG inactivation. Channel availability decreases at positive potentials resulting in the bell-shaped *I–V* relationship. From Sanguinetti (2010) *Pflugers Arch.* **460**, 265–276 with permission.

in the *I–V* relationship being bell-shaped, almost mirroring the behaviour of the L-type Ca^{2+} channel *I–V* relation (Fig. 7.4).

Voltage clamp experiments illustrate the unusual behaviour of the channels. As cardiac myocytes are clamped to more positive potentials the current at the end of the clamp step increases much like other voltage-gated K^+ channels. When the cells are repolarized to a negative holding potential the amplitudes of the currents suddenly become much larger and then decay *unlike* other delayed rectifier voltage-gated K^+ channels. These are so-called "tail currents", a name given to currents that flow after the voltage clamp step. Tail currents are caused by channels that initially, during the depolarization, have activated. As the depolarization step continues these channels inactivate and when the membrane is repolarized the channels rapidly recover from the inactivation. At more positive clamp step potentials the inactivation is greater so that, following repolarization, more channels recover producing larger tails. Once the membrane potential is clamped back to (near) rest the current decay follows the time course of channel deactivation. The maximum size of the tail currents immediately after the voltage step is dependent on the number of channels re-opening and on the driving force on the ion. The decay of tail currents gives information about the time course of the deactivation process.

The unusually rapid inactivation is due to a voltage-dependent C-type inactivation process (see Chapter 6, p. 146) which limits K^+ flow at positive voltages.

The difference between the membrane potential during phase 2 and the voltage dependence of activation of the channels governs the extent of current flow during the plateau and later the number of channels recovering from inactivation governs the amount of current. The maximum I_{Kr} amplitude during the action potential is relatively small compared with I_{K1}, but it plays a major role bringing about an end to the plateau (phase 2) and initiating phase 3.

7.3.3 I_{Kr} and hERG

Similar, but not identical behaviour to I_{Kr} was observed in groups of mutant K^+ channels expressed in *Drosophila* (see Chapter 4, pp. 73–74). Flies expressing this form of K^+ channel had the behavioural characteristic of moving like a go-go dancer following exposure to ether due to a high level of spontaneous activity in the motor nerves serving their skeletal muscles. This form of channel therefore became known as the ether-a-go-go (or EAG) channel. A few years later, the human form of this channel type was cloned and this, naturally, became known as the human ether-a-go-go related gene (or hERG) channel. The hERG channel is closely related to the EAG channels but with some fundamental differences in function. EAG produces a delayed rectifier current that does not inactivate and probably plays a role in neuro-muscular transmission and controlling the cell cycle, whereas hERG produces the voltage-gated potassium channel with rapid C-type inactivation and inwardly rectifying properties. When hERG channels are experimentally expressed in oocytes that usually lack them, the current produced has many of the features of I_{Kr}. Though often treated as essentially synonymous, the term "hERG" should be used when discussing the molecularly engineered channel because this does not have modulatory subunits associated with it. The term "I_{Kr}" is used when talking about the rapid delayed rectifier current that arises as a result of hERG channels and their associated subunits.

I_{Kr} flows through the $K_{V11.1}$ (hERG) potassium ion channel coded by the gene KCNH2. The closely related EAG channels belong to the $K_{V10.1}$ subfamily and are coded by the gene KCNH1. The channel has the typical K_V family structure of a tetrameric complex of four α-subunits. In expression systems hERG channels produce currents with slightly different activation and inactivation characteristics compared with currents in normal heart cells. This suggests that, in the native cell types, other channel subunits associate with $K_{V11.1}$ channels modulating their properties. The main candidate is MinK-related protein (MiRP1), a 123 amino acid protein with a single membrane-spanning domain encoded by the KCNE2 gene. When co-expressed with hERG, MiRP1 shifts the I_{Kr} activation curve to more positive potentials and accelerates the rate of current deactivation. Another accessory subunit that can also modify hERG function is called MinK but this subunit seems to play a much more important role in the modulation of I_{Ks} (see p. 197). The methanesulphonanilides (e.g. E-4031 and dofetilide) are specific inhibitors of the $K_{V11.1}$ channel with respective K_d of around 8 and 4 nM.

They block the channels by binding when they are open but it is not certain to what channel structure they bind.

7.3.3.1 *hERG and long QT syndrome*

$K_{V11.1}$ (hERG) forms the major portion of an important K^+ channel that allows K^+ ions to flow out of cardiac myocytes causing their repolarization. If the function of this channel is inhibited or compromised, either by drugs or genetic mutation, the cell action potential duration prolongs. In the whole heart, the repolarization process is lengthened, increasing the QT interval on the ECG, hence such disorders produce "drug-induced" (also known as "acquired") and "genetic" long QT syndrome.

Following independent descriptions in the 1960s by an Italian paediatrician, Cesarino Romano, and his colleagues and an Irish doctor, Owen Ward, of patients who had episodes of syncope followed by sudden death, it was gradually realized that ventricular arrhythmias linked with long QT intervals were their underlying cause and that the clinical problem could be inherited. Better clinical descriptions of the Romano–Ward syndrome were obtained along with genetic screening of patients while, in parallel, there was rapid progress made on identifying the molecular characteristics of many ion channels. It is now known that mutated forms of $K_{V11.1}$ (and $K_{V7.1}$ – see p. 197) can cause some of the inherited forms of long QT syndrome (LQTS). Over 450 mutations in the coding gene KCNH2 have now been described and these translate into a variety of functional abnormalities of the channel protein, from disrupted trafficking to mis-folding and sequence deletions. These all cause a loss of channel function which leads to abnormal repolarization of the cardiac myocytes and differences in their refractory periods. Epicardial myocytes can express different amounts of I_{Kr} compared with endocardial myocytes. Therefore, patients with these mutations will exhibit a large range of action potential durations amongst their myocytes with heterogeneous repolarization times and refractory periods. This situation is termed "increased *dispersion* of APD". If there are regions of the heart with longer refractory periods compared with other closely neighbouring areas, this presents opportunities for re-excitation of the regions before the normal, rhythmical excitatory event occurs. Such re-excitation can start so-called re-entrant arrhythmias. This is discussed in more detail in the Chapter 9.

In addition, the longer APDs observed in these patients can predispose the myocytes to after-depolarizations which also are pro-arrhythmic. Early after-depolarizations are due to re-opening of L-type Ca^{2+} channels during the plateau phase of the action potential. As detailed in Chapter 6, adrenergic stimulation increases the open time of these channels, which leads to further depolarization and more arrhythmias. This is one explanation for an increased risk of sudden death in individuals with LQTS during exercise or following periods of agitation or excitement when their adrenergic drive is greater than normal. Better genetic testing can identify ion channel mutations more precisely and this has lead to a more exact system of nomenclature, as detailed in Table 7.1.

$K_{V11.1}$ is very susceptible to blockade from a variety of drugs – much more than other K_V channels. This suggests that the structure of the channel, although fundamentally typical for the K_V family, has a different configuration that allows some drugs to block ion access to the selectivity pore relatively easily. Compounds that block the channel are very diverse in structure yet can be remarkably selective for $K_{V11.1}$ over other ion channels. Such high affinity compounds tend to block only when the channel is open. These observations together suggest that (1) the channel gates provide an initial barrier to drugs gaining access to the selectivity pore and (2) there is likely to be a larger than normal vestibule that accommodates assorted forms of blocking agents which then impede access to the conduction pore itself. "Drug trapping" and molecular biology studies point to two structural features of $K_{V11.1}$ not shared by other voltage-gated K_V channels which are probably responsible for these promiscuous drug interactions.

Firstly, the channel lacks proline residues in the S6 trans-membrane domain (Table 7.2). This Pro-X-Pro sequence (where the X is an unspecified amino acid) is normally highly conserved in K_{VX} channels and is and is thought to induce a kink in the S6 domain. The kink allows

Long QT form	Mutation site	Current affected	Gene affected	Comments
LQT1	α-subunit of $K_{V7.1}$ (K_{VLQT1})	I_{Ks}	KCNQ1	Mutations decrease I_{Ks}. Commonest but least severe.
LQT2	α-subunit of $K_{V11.1}$	I_{Kr}	KCNH2	Mutations decrease I_{Kr}.
LQT3	α-subunit of $Na_{V1.5}$	I_{Na}	SCN5A	Small Na^+ influx continues until late in the action potential due to some channels failing to inactivate normally. Severe phenotype but less common.
LQT4	Ankyrin B	various	ANK2	Ankyrin B anchors and helps orientate channels and transporters in cell membranes. Rare form.
LQT5	β-subunit of MinK	I_{Ks}	KCNE1	Co-assembles with $K_{V7.1}$.
LQT6	β-subunit of MiRP1	I_{Kr}	KCNE2	Co-assembles with $K_{V11.1}$ (hERG).
LQT7	α-subunit of $K_{ir2.1}$	I_{K1}	KCNJ2	Changes function of $K_{ir2.1}$ or affects trafficking or insertion of protein into membrane. Andersen–Tawil syndrome.
LQT8	α-subunit of $Ca_{V1.2}$	$I_{Ca,L}$	CACNA1C	Delays channel inactivation prolonging depolarizing current. Timothy syndrome.
LQT9	Caveolin-3	various	CAV3	Scaffolding proteins for organizing and trafficking channels into membrane

Table 7.1. Nomenclature of LQT syndromes.

LQT10	β-subunit of Na$_{V1.5}$	I_{Na}	SCN4B	Na$_{Vβ4}$ is a β-subunit of Na$_{v1.5}$. Mutation causes rightward (+ve) shift in inactivation relationship.
LQT11	AKAP (A-kinase anchor protein)	unknown	AKAP9	AKAPs bind to regulatory subunit of PKA affecting cellular distribution of enzyme.
LQT12	α-1-syntrophin	? I_{Na}	SNTA1	PDZ domain of α-1-syntrophin may regulate Na$_{V1.5}$. α-1-syntrophin is a form of dystrophin, a cytoskeletal protein missing in patients with Duchenne's muscular dystrophy.
LQT13	Subunit forming K$_{ir3.4}$ (GIRK4)	$I_{Kir3.4}$, (I_{GIRK})	KCNJ5	

Table 7.1. (Continued).

the lower half of the S6 to move and angles it towards the S4–S5 linker. The lack of the Pro-X-Pro sequence removes the kink and makes the S6 domain more flexible and capable of forming a larger inner vestibule (Fig. 7.5).

Secondly, the presence of two aromatic residues, tyrosine and phenylalanine (Y and F) (Tyr652 and Phe656), in the same domain seem to be important for drug binding (Fig. 7.5). The drugs appear to block the channel by crossing the surface membrane and entering from the cytoplasmic side. Provided the channel is open the drugs have access to binding sites in the larger than normal central cavity. When the channel closes, structural modifications around the binding site take place so that drugs that are small enough can fit into the closed vestibule.

Channel	Conserved S6 sequence
$K_{V1.1}$	AGVLTIAL**P**V**P**VIV
$K_{V1.5}$	AGVLTIAL**P**V**P**VIV
$K_{V2.1}$	AGVLVIAL**P**V**P**VII
$K_{V3.1}$	AGVLTIAM**P**V**P**VIV
$K_{V4.1}$	SGVLVIAL**P**V**P**VIV
$K_{V4.2}$	SGVLTIAL**P**V**P**VIV
$K_{V4.3}$	SGVLVIAL**P**V**P**VIV
hERG	IGSLM**Y**ASI**F**GNVS

Table 7.2. Amino acid sequence in S6.

Larger compounds prevent the channel from closing completely and so they can dissociate from the channel in a (nearly) closed state – termed the "foot in the door" mechanism. Principally for these structural reasons, a large number of diverse compounds bind to $K_{V11.1}$ blocking the channel and so greatly increase the risk of potentially fatal cardiac arrhythmias. QT interval prolongation is a major safety concern of drug regulatory bodies and pharmaceutical companies invest heavily in making sure compounds under development do not have this undesirable side effect. It is estimated that at least half of all new "pipeline" drugs are found to block $K_{V11.1}$ channels. Development of these drugs generally then ceases at that point.

7.3.4 I_{Ks}

I_{Ks} is also a delayed rectifier current and gradually increases as the cells depolarize. The channel type through which I_{Ks} flows is $K_{V7.1}$ (also known as K_{VLQT1}) and the gene that codes the protein is KCNQ1. The channel is voltage gated. It shows very slow activation on depolarization but plays a role in determining the later plateau amplitude, the initial phase of faster repolarization at the end of phase 2 and the start of phase 3. It therefore can affect action potential shape and duration. The time constant for activation of I_{Ks} is dependent on species but is in the range 250–450 ms, so the current is never fully activated at normal heart rates. $K_{V7.1}$ channels have a small single-channel conductance in the range of a

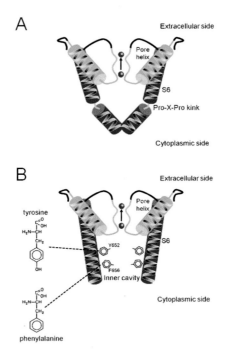

Figure 7.5.   Two structural features of $K_{V11.1}$ responsible for drug interactions. Panel A shows the structure of a typical Kv channel.   The Pro-X-Pro sequence is thought to induce a kink in the S6 domain producing a smaller inner cavity.   Panel B shows the structure of a $K_{V11.1}$ channel.   The lack of Pro-X-Pro sequence removes the kink and allows a larger inner cavity to be formed.   The two aromatic residues, tyrosine and phenylalanine (Y652 and F656) appear important for drug binding.

few picosiemens. They vary in density across the ventricular wall – being less in the midmyocardial cell layer than in epi- or endocardium – and greater in the base than the apex, so the longest APD is measured in apical M cells. Therefore the expression of I_{Ks} is thought to play a large role in determining the transmural dispersion of APD.

The channel is composed of the standard K^+ channel tetramer with about 600 amino acid residues and the voltage sensor located in S4. Normally during the action potential I_{Ks} would not inactivate appreciably but on longer depolarizing steps under voltage clamp a fraction of the channels show some inactivation. The inactivation property stems from parts of the protein in the S5 and pore loop domains because changes of a single residue in these parts of the molecule can abolish the process. Channel deactivation is also slow (the process has two components, fast and slow, with time constants about 200 and 700 ms respectively) so I_{Ks} tends to build at high heart rates because less time is available for it to deactivate completely before another action potential. Following another depolarization there will be more channels in the active state. This "accumulation" of I_{Ks} also appears to occur in the presence of β-adrenergic agonists.

Additionally, at faster heart rates the kinetics of I_{Ks} activation are also accelerated and so the current is greater when stimulation rate increases. The most probable explanation for this effect is that, at the end of the diastolic interval, more $K_{V7.1}$ channels may be in a transitional state towards full activation compared with the situation at lower heart rates. Conversion from this to the final open state would then be faster. Sanguinetti and colleagues found that the deactivation rate was inversely proportional to the duration of the activating step, so it would be likely that more channels were in the transitional state when the ratio between action potential duration and diastolic interval is increased, as occurs at shorter cycle lengths.

The role of I_{Ks} in repolarization remains controversial. Some findings indicate that pharmacological inhibition of the current does not affect APD while others find an expected prolongation. Mutation of the channel produces long QT intervals. Pharmacological inhibition of I_{Ks} has a greater effect on APD if the action potential is already prolonged. This is mainly because more I_{Ks} is activated during a long action potential. This property of the current may confer the myocardial cells with a "repolarization reserve" that acts to limit excessive APD prolongation which can be arrhythmogenic. Chromanol 293B is a selective blocker of I_{Ks} ($K_d = 1$ μM) and appears to bind in the central cavity of the channel interacting with residues Ile337 and Phe340 and the selectivity filter.

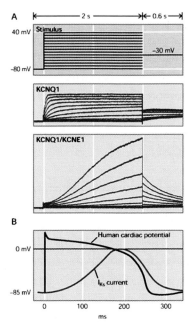

Figure 7.6.   Typical characteristics of I_{Ks}. Panel A illustrates the voltage clamp protocol used to elicit the currents shown in the lower traces. Steps to increasingly more positive voltages are followed by a step back to a partially depolarized voltage of –30 mV. The responses to this protocol of the α-subunit alone (KCNQ1) and the α- and β-subunit co-expressed (KCNQ1/KCNE1) are shown.   The subunits were expressed in HEK (human embryonic kidney) 293 cells. Panel B illustrates when I_{Ks} would flow during a human cardiac action potential. From Jespersen *et al.* (2005) *Physiology* **20**, 408–416.

Although KCNQ1 alone produces tetrameric units that form functional voltage-gated channels (the α-subunits), these tend to activate rapidly and reach a maximum current during a large depolarizing voltage clamp step. A fully functional channel complex that replicates the kinetic properties of I_{Ks} requires the co-assembly of the α-subunit with the β-subunit coded by the gene KCNE1 (Fig. 7.6). This gene codes for a protein called "minK", one of five members of a KCNE family of proteins, which is also known as the "minimal K^+ channel" subunit. All the KCNE-derived subunits are small proteins with one trans-membrane spanning region and an extracellular NH_2 terminal. minK was cloned in 1988 and was so-called because injection of its cDNA into *Xenopus* oocytes produced a small and slow current that had some similar properties to I_{Ks}. However, comparable transfection of minK cDNA into mammalian expression systems somewhat puzzlingly failed to produce a current, and it was not until $K_{V7.1}$ (and its gene KCNQ1) was found that it was realized that the currents originally recorded in *Xenopus* oocytes arose from the co-assembly of endogenously expressed $K_{V7.1}$ and the newly expressed minK subunits. The minK subunit binds to the outer part of the $K_{V7.1}$ pore loop from where it modulates channel function. Mutations in either KCNQ1 or KCNE1 can cause congenital long QT syndromes.

7.3.5 Na^+/Ca^{2+} exchange

As mentioned in Chapter 5, the Na^+/Ca^{2+} exchange is electrogenic, with the direction of the net charge movement varying depending on membrane potential, intracellular $[Na^+]$ and intracellular $[Ca^{2+}]$. The direction the exchange transports these ions can be predicted from knowing its reversal potential (E_{rev}) calculated using Eqn. 5.2.

At membrane potentials more positive than E_{rev}, the exchange will carry Ca^{2+} into the cell and Na^+ will be expelled. Conversely, at membrane potentials more negative than E_{rev}, the exchange will carry Na^+ into the cell and Ca^{2+} will be moved out. During phase 2 of the action potential the cytoplasmic $[Ca^{2+}]$ is greater than at rest because Ca^{2+} has just been released from the SR forming the Ca^{2+} transient and this increase in $[Ca^{2+}]$ forces E_{rev} in the positive direction. The operation of the exchange therefore produces net inward current, expelling Ca^{2+} as Na^+ is transported into the cell. It remains in this forward mode for phase 2 and phase 3 as it helps expel a portion of the Ca^{2+} that contributes to the transient. In fact, the exchanger is the main Ca^{2+} efflux pathway in cells and is responsible for removing the same amount of Ca^{2+} as enters the cell during L-type Ca^{2+} current activation in phase 1, so maintaining balanced Ca^{2+} entry and exit. The relative importance of the exchange as a Ca^{2+} efflux system varies between species. In human it probably contributes about 20–25% to Ca^{2+} removal from the cytoplasm (with by far the largest contribution coming from the SR Ca^{2+}ATPase) but in rat and mouse its contribution is much less – probably near 5–10%. The inward current of about 2–3 A.F^{-1} produced by the efflux of Ca^{2+} helps sustain the plateau depolarization near the end of phase 2 as the K$^+$ currents (I_{Kr} and I_{Ks}) become more activated. Thus the exchange plays a role in determining the APD and couples the APD to the Ca^{2+} transient.

In phase 0 during the upstroke of the action potential, the membrane potential very quickly becomes more positive than E_{rev} before there is substantial Ca^{2+} release from the SR and so the exchanger current is very briefly outward. This so-called reverse mode of the exchange may provide another route for Ca^{2+} entry into the cells at the very start of the action potential, but the physiological relevance of this Ca^{2+} influx is controversial. Calculating the precise time course of the inward and reverse modes of the exchanger during the cardiac cycle is more complex than it appears because, although we can make reasonable estimates of cytoplasmic Ca^{2+}, accurately modelling the behaviour of the exchange relies on knowing the sub-sarcolemmal [Ca^{2+}] near the ion binding sites of the protein itself. It is this concentration that influences E_{rev} and probably differs from the cytoplasmic [Ca^{2+}] because of restricted diffusion in the microdomain of the dyadic cleft where the exchange is mainly located. We lack reliable techniques for the measurement of Ca^{2+} in this space.

The contribution that the exchange makes to early Ca^{2+} influx and phase 2 and phase 3 Ca^{2+} efflux changes greatly when intracellular [Na$^+$] increases (which can occur as a result of increased rate of stimulation, Na$^+$/K$^+$ pump inhibition or hypoxia). Intracellular [Na$^+$] only requires to change by several millimoles to markedly alter the time the exchange spends in either inward or reverse mode during one cardiac cycle, and this ultimately influences APD and the size and duration of the Ca^{2+} transient.

Since the exchange modulates intracellular [Ca^{2+}] and therefore cell contractility, it would seem an ideal drug target for inotropic interventions, particularly if its activity could be selectively and directionally controlled. However, to date there are very few drugs that change its operation specifically. Amiloride and derivatives such as 3′-4′-dichlorobenzamil have been used as inhibitors of the exchange, but they are not potent (K_d of several millimolar) and have a variety of non-specific actions. A more recent derivative, KB-R7943, has a higher potency (K_d approx. 10 μM) but still is not selective at this concentration, affecting a variety of ion channels notably those carrying Ca^{2+} and K^+. A compound called SEA-0400 (2-[4-[(2,5-difluorophenyl)methoxy]-phenoxy]-5-ethoxyaniline) also inhibits $I_{Ca,L}$ with micromolar affinity but it appears to be much more potent than KB-R7943 in inhibiting the exchange with an approximate K_d of 0.11 μM.

7.3.6 $I_{Na,late}$

In the previous chapter it was emphasized that almost all Na^+ channels inactivate within a few milliseconds of the start of the action potential and the channels remain in that state for the duration of the plateau, only becoming available again in phase 3. Since inactivation is time dependent, the cells then enter a refractory period during which another stimulation pulse will fail to open the inactivated channels.

For reasons that are not understood a small percentage of Na^+ channels either (1) fail to enter an inactivated state and remain open or (2) inactivate, close and then re-open during the action potential. These channels carry a Na^+ current that, although very small (usually <1% of the peak of I_{Na}), persists throughout the plateau and so has been termed $I_{Na,p}$ (p for persistent) or $I_{Na,late}$ (Fig. 7.7). The channels through which $I_{Na,late}$ flows remain to be precisely characterized, but the majority of the current flows through the same type of channels that carry I_{Na} ($Na_{V1.5}$) since it can be recorded in expression systems when only $Na_{V1.5}$ channels are present. These may have some different properties from the normal $Na_{V1.5}$ channels that are not fully understood. The current is inhibited by local anaesthetics and TTX at the usual high concentrations seen in cardiac tissue. The late Na^+ current, though very small compared with the extremely large, brief fast Na^+ current (<0.1 A.F^{-1} cf. 250 A.F^{-1}), allows a sustained influx of Na^+ into the cells throughout the action potential that is sufficient to prolong APD (Fig. 7.7). Influx of Na^+ by this route may be quite large because, although the current is small, it flows for a

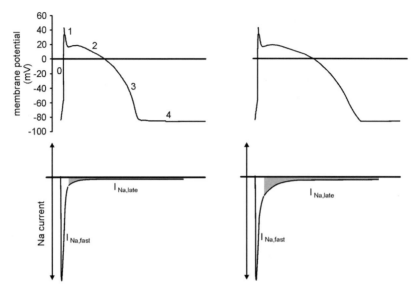

Figure 7.7. The relationship between the "classic" I_{Na} that produces the action potential upstroke (here designated as $I_{Na,fast}$) and the late Na^+ current (designated as $I_{Na,late}$) and shaded. In the right panel, $I_{Na,late}$ has increased without the peak of the $I_{Na,fast}$ changing. This increased $I_{Na,late}$ causes a prolongation of the plateau and action potential duration.

long period so that its integral is of a similar value to the brief early current surge. Lidocaine and TTX application shorten APD potentially via a reduction in $I_{Na,late}$.

Whilst we know that $Na_{V1.5}$ has a low sensitivity to TTX and STX, Cd^{2+} also appears to inhibit the late Na^+ current, producing a 50% block around 100 μM. The most specific blocker that is also currently in clinical use is ranolazine, which preferentially blocks $I_{Na,late}$ over the normal early I_{Na} by 10 to 40 times (6 μM vs 250 μM). However, ranolazine is not completely specific in this context because it also blocks I_{Kr} at about double the concentration at which it blocks $I_{Na,late}$.

$I_{Na,late}$ may play a role in cardiac arrhythmogenesis. It has been shown that a genetic mutation in $Na_{V1.5}$ produces inadequate inactivation of the channel. Patients with this congenital defect have LQT3 syndrome resulting from a gain of function effect on the channel. Prolongation of the action potential is a common finding in myocytes isolated from failing hearts. The main cause of this prolongation is a decrease in function of K^+ channels – mainly those carrying I_{to} – and this leads to a decrease in speed of repolarization with a "loss of function" effect. Recent work has indicated that cells isolated from failing hearts may also have larger $I_{Na,late}$, which would prolong depolarization and hence increase ADP due to a "gain of function" effect.

7.4 Phase 3

As repolarization proceeds and the membrane potential becomes more negative, the inward rectifying channels producing I_{K1} tend to open again at potentials negative to –20 mV. The size of I_{K1} becomes larger as the membrane repolarizes more and phase 3, the termination of the plateau and final cell repolarization, is essentially entirely due to I_{K1}. I_{K1} then continues to flow so stabilizing the resting membrane potential. $I_{Na/Ca}$ also becomes larger during this phase because intracellular $[Ca^{2+}]$ is still raised and the more negative membrane potential (compared with the end of phase 2) increases the forward mode exchange current. It is important to note that diastolic intracellular $[Ca^{2+}]$ is not reached until some time after the action potential has completely repolarized. Once the resting membrane potential has been reached it is held at that value by a continuous flow of outward I_{K1}. This is large enough to keep membrane potential stable even though $I_{Na/Ca}$ is still producing inward current whilst expelling residual Ca^{2+} from the cell.

7.5 A summary of repolarizing currents

A number of K^+ channels are involved in repolarizing heart cells and therefore in determining the duration of the action potential. These are summarized in Table 7.3.

Current	Channel(s)	Gene	Activator
$I_{to1,f}$	$K_{V4.2}/K_{V4.3}$	KCND2/3	Depolarization
$I_{to1,s}$	$K_{V1.4}$	KCNA4	Depolarization
I_{to2}	ClCA1	TMEM16	[Ca]
I_{Kur}	$K_{V1.5}$	KCNA5	Depolarization
I_{Kr}	$K_{V11.1}$	KCNH2	Depolarization
I_{Ks}	$K_{V7.1}$	KCNQ1	Depolarization
I_{K1}	$K_{ir2.1}/K_{ir2.2}$	KCNJ2/12	Depolarization
I_{KACh}	$K_{ir3.1}/K_{ir3.4}$	KCNJ3/5	Acetylcholine
I_{KATP}	$K_{ir6.2}$	KCNJ11	[ADP]:[ATP] Plus SUR2A coded by ABCC9 gene

Table 7.3. A summary of repolarizing currents.

7.6 Questions

(1) Describe the *I–V* relationship of I_{K1}. What is the main molecular mechanism that underlies the anomalous behaviour of this current?

(2) What happens to I_{K1} in hyperkalaemia and what consequences does this have for conduction in the myocardium?

(3) Explain why I_{Kur} might be an effective target for selective drug therapy for atrial fibrillation.

(4) What structural features of $K_{V11.1}$ not shared by other voltage-gated K_V channels are thought to be responsible for its large number of drug interactions?

(5) Explain why slow Ca^{2+} release from the SR might prolong the action potential.

7.7 Bibliography

7.7.1 *Reviews*

Hibino, H., Inanobe, A., Furutani, K. *et al.* (2010). Inwardly rectifying potassium channels: their structure, function, and physiological roles. *Physiol. Rev.* **90**, 291–366.

Jespersen, T., Grunnet, M. and Olesen, S.-P. (2005). The KCNQ1 potassium channel: from gene to physiological function. *Physiology* **20**, 408–416.

Lopatin, A.N. and Nichols, C.G. (2001). Inward rectifiers in the heart: an update on I_{K1}. *J. Mol. Cell. Cardiol.* **33**, 625–638.

Maltsev, V.A. and Undrovinas, A. (2008). Late sodium current in failing heart: friend or foe? *Prog. Biophys. Mol. Biol.* **96**, 421–451.

Ravens, U. and Wettwer, E. (2011). Ultra-rapid delayed rectifier channels: molecular basis and therapeutic implications. *Cardiovasc. Res.* **89**, 776–785.

Sanguinetti, M.C. (2010). HERG1 channelopathies. *Pflugers Arch.* **460**, 265–276.

7.7.2 *Original papers*

Kurata, H.T., Phillips, L.R., Rose, T. *et al.* (2004). Molecular basis of inward rectification: polyamine interaction sites located by combined channel and ligand mutagenesis. *J. Gen. Physiol.* **124**, 541–554.

Maltsev, V.A., Sabbah, H.N., Higgins, R.S.D. *et al.* (1998). Novel, ultraslow inactivating sodium current in human ventricular cardiomyocytes. *Circulation* **98**, 2545–2552.

Sakmann, B. and Trube, G. (1984). Conductance properties on single inwardly rectifiying potassium channels in ventricular cells from guinea-pig heart. *J. Physiol.* **347**, 641–657.

Chapter 8

Ionic Basis of Automaticity

Different parts of the heart have distinct action potential shapes largely as a consequence of variations in the expression of ionic channels and other membrane transport mechanisms. It would be too time consuming to provide detailed descriptions of the currents flowing in all other cardiac cell types and this would detract from the central emphasis of the book, which is to provide an introduction to cardiac cell electrophysiology. The intention of this chapter is to describe the main currents flowing in cells from the sino-atrial (or sinu-atrial) node. This will allow the reader to (1) compare and contrast the differences with a ventricular myocyte in terms of duration of action potential and function of the ionic channels and (2) understand how pacemaking occurs.

8.1   Chapter objectives

After reading this chapter you should be able to:

- Understand that cardiac myocytes isolated from various parts of the heart have different action potential shapes largely as a consequence of variations in the expression of ionic channels and other membrane transport mechanisms
- Describe the pacemaker current, I_f, in terms of activation and sensitivity to the neurotransmitters acetylcholine and noradrenaline
- Discuss the influence of $I_{Ca,T}$ on the sino-atrial nodal cell action potential
- Explain the alternative "Ca^{2+} clock" hypothesis of pacemaking

8.2 The sino-atrial node

The sino-atrial (SA) node lies at the anterior and superior margins of the groove that forms the boundary between the right atrium and the superior vena cava. The node is a spindle or tear-drop shaped structure that usually lies just below the epicardial surface. From there it runs more deeply to join cardiac myocytes belonging to the right atrium. At its centre are the main pacemaker cells termed "P" cells. They are between 5 and 10 µm in diameter, 20 to 30 µm in length, and have so few myofibrils that it is debatable whether or not they are muscle cells. There are comparatively few gap junctions in this area leading some to suggest that the junctions are located in key areas to produce preferential conduction pathways for action potential propagation from the centre.

As the nodal cells spread there is a transition in their morphology and architecture towards the periphery of the node where the cells meet atrial myocytes. The cells become larger, have more defined myofilaments and contain more mitochondria. This transitional zone is interspersed with connective tissue which may guide conduction through certain routes, but the pathways for impulse exit from the node are poorly understood. Although there is some heterogeneity of action potential shape across the node (reflecting subtle differences in ion channel expression), essentially all SA nodal cells show the slow diastolic depolarization during phase 4 that is their characteristic hallmark (Fig. 8.1A).

The slow depolarization illustrates that SA nodal cells have an unstable resting membrane potential and this instability arises from a lack of I_{K1}. Remember from Chapter 7 (pp. 180–182) that near E_K the conductance of this channel is high (the membrane is very permeable to K^+) so other currents need to be large to change the membrane potential. Therefore, cells with I_{K1} tend to have stable resting (phase 4) membrane potentials. With no I_{K1}, SA nodal cells have a much lower resting membrane conductance so that small changes in currents flowing across the membrane can produce large changes in membrane potential. So, while the unstable membrane potential arises from a lack of I_{K1}, how can the slow depolarization be explained? The slow depolarization is due to the decay of an outward current and an increase in various inward currents. We will begin with describing one of the inward currents, the importance of which is underlined by it often being called "the pacemaker current".

8.3 I_f

In 1976 Noma and Irisawa recorded, in voltage-clamped rabbit SA nodal preparations, an inward current that had the unusual characteristic of becoming larger as the preparation was *hyperpolarized*. In the discussion section of their paper they noted, "It appears difficult to explain the inward current changes during and after the hyperpolarizing pulses" and they remained puzzled about its origin. This unusual current behaviour was observed again and more clearly described three years later by Hilary Brown, Dario DiFrancesco and Susan Noble who called the current I_f and noted that it was modulated by adrenaline.

The peculiar behaviour of the current in response to voltage changes and the fact that it could be carried by Na^+ and K^+ ions gave rise to the term "funny current" (I_f). Largely through the continued work of DiFrancesco, the current in the heart is now well described and has many features appropriate for its role as the main pacemaker current. It activates slowly on hyperpolarization from around –45 mV (Fig. 8.1B) with a time constant of activation of about 500 ms, deactivates rapidly upon depolarization to more positive voltages, is increased by β-receptor stimulation and inhibited by acetylcholine (Fig. 8.2). These properties help in the generation of a slowly developing diastolic depolarization that can be modulated by neurotransmitters.

The potential at which I_f reverses is about –25 mV so the current is inward (and carried by Na^+) near the maximum diastolic potential reached by the SA nodal cells (i.e. at voltages more negative than the reversal potential) and outward (carried by K^+) at depolarized membrane potentials more positive than the reversal potential. As the maximum diastolic potential is reached, more channels carrying I_f become activated resulting in a progressive increase in depolarizing current. As the diastolic depolarization phase progresses to more positive potentials

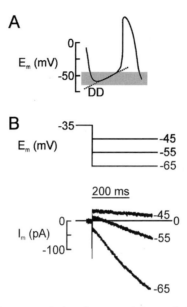

Figure 8.1.   Panel A shows a typical action potential recorded from an isolated rabbit sino-atrial cell.   Note the slow diastolic depolarization (DD).   The shaded rectangle indicates the range of voltages (between –45 and –65 mV) used in the voltage clamp experiment illustrated in Panel B.   Panel B shows current traces recorded in the same cell type during voltage clamp steps to the levels indicated from a holding potential of 35 mV. Redrawn from DiFrancesco (1991) *J. Physiol.* **434**, 23–40.

fewer funny channels remain activated because depolarization deactivates the channels and the size of the current gradually declines.

As I_f became better described, it was realized that it had shared characteristics with currents in the brain and retina (there called I_h – for hyperpolarizing) that flowed through the <u>H</u>yperpolarization-activated <u>C</u>yclic <u>N</u>ucleotide-gated (or HCN) group of channels.

8.3.1 *HCN channels*

HCN channels in the heart belong to a family comprising four members (HCN1–HCN4) each with about 60% sequence homology to the others. HCN4 is the main isoform expressed in the SA node, though small numbers of HCN1 and HCN2 channels have been reported. The isoforms

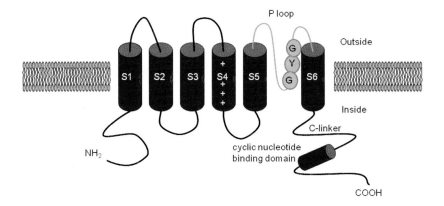

Figure 8.2. The structure of a monomer of HCN channels.

differ in their speed of activation (HCN1 is the most rapidly activated and HCN4 the slowest) and the extent to which they are modulated by cAMP (HCN2 and 4 producing the largest voltage shift in their activation curves for a given [cAMP]). HCN4 channels are formed from four identical (but sometimes non-identical) segments each with six trans-membrane domains. The S4 segments of the tetramers serve as the voltage sensors while the C-terminals of the assembled protein are attached to a cyclic nucleotide binding domain that allows the channel to be regulated primarily by cyclic AMP. The cyclic nucleotide binding domain is connected to the sixth trans-membrane domain by a short stretch of protein called the C-linker.

The P loop of each monomer has a GYG (glycine, tyrosine, glycine) grouping of amino acid residues which, as in many other types of K^+ channel, constitutes the selectivity filter. However, HCN channels are also permeable to Na^+ ions so their inner pore is probably less rigid than that of other K^+ channels and this allows partially hydrated Na^+ ions to pass through. Whilst there are obvious similarities in structure between HCN and K^+ channels, there are profound differences in the way the channels react to trans-membrane voltage changes. HCN channels open with hyperpolarization whereas K^+ channels open with depolarization, so the way the voltage sensors and associated proteins react to a voltage change probably involves opposite coupling mechanisms, but the mechanism is not known. Single alanine substitutions of the S4–S5 linker disrupts channel closing suggesting the linker is involved in channel gating. The S4–S5 link region may also electrostatically interact with the C-linker region stabilizing the closed state of the channel and effectively coupling voltage sensing to channel gating.

The HCN channel open probability is modulated by innervation from the autonomic nervous system. In isolated SA node cells, the presence of β-receptor agonists increases the rate of diastolic depolarization and the presence of acetylcholine (ACh) slows the rate (Fig. 8.3). The binding of cyclic AMP is not required for channel activation *per se* nor is channel conductance altered. Rather, cyclic AMP shifts the voltage dependence of channel activation to more positive membrane potentials and thereby increases the number of open channels at a given voltage (Fig. 8.4). This increases the number of channels through which depolarizing current flows and so the rate of depolarization becomes faster which, in turn, allows heart rate to increase (Fig. 8.3). Conversely, when ACh binds to muscarinic receptors on the cell membrane, adenylate cyclase activity is suppressed by an inhibitory G-protein and the production of cAMP decreases. With less cAMP, the activation curve shifts leftwards to more negative potentials and thereby decreases the number of open channels at a given voltage. Under these conditions less depolarizing current flows and so the rate of depolarization is slower (Fig. 8.3).

Crystallization experiments have shown that cAMP binding alters the conformation of the C-linkers with respect to each other, "locking" the channels in an open state. This effect is the result of a direct interaction of intracellular cAMP with the channels and is not dependent upon phosphorylation. The C-linker and cyclic nucleotide binding domain seem to be an auto-inhibitory component of the channel. If the [cAMP] is low, the auto-inhibition component inhibits channel gating probably by blocking the channel pore, with the result that the activation curve shifts leftwards. If the cAMP concentration increases, the auto-inhibition is relieved and the voltage dependence of channel activation shifts to the right (Fig. 8.4).

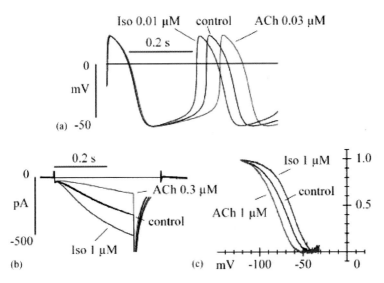

Figure 8.3. The gradient of the diastolic depolarization is dependent on the actions of autonomic nervous system transmitters. Upper panel designated (a): Isoprenaline (blue trace) accelerates and acetylcholine (red trace) slows the spontaneous rate in isolated SAN cells. Lower panel, part (b): Isoprenaline (blue trace) increases and acetylcholine (red trace) decreases I_f produced by voltage clamp steps from −35 to −85 mV. Lower panel, part (c): The effects of the transmitters cause right (isoprenaline − blue) and left (acetylcholine − red) shifts of the activation curve of I_f. Reproduced from DiFrancesco (2006) *Pharmacol. Res.* **53**, 399–406 with permission.

The HCN channels can associate with a β-subunit, MinK-related protein 1 (MiRP1 or KCNE2) and such an interaction increases current density. As might be expected, the current density and HCN expression level is greatest in SA nodal tissue and less elsewhere in the heart. The I_f density in human SA nodal cells is about −8 pA.pF^{-1} but the density decreases to about −0.8 and −0.5 pA.pF^{-1} in human atrial and ventricular myocytes respectively. In the ventricle, its range of activation is also more negative than in the SA node (lying between −80 and −120 mV) so the current is unlikely to have any functional role in the atria and ventricles. It is present in the atrioventricular node and in Purkinje fibres but what role it performs in those tissues is uncertain.

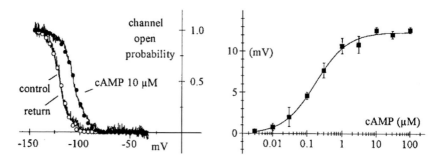

Figure 8.4. Left panel: Plots of the funny channel open probability (P_o) measured using the inside-out patch method on a SA nodal cell, firstly in control solution, then during and after superfusion of the intracellular side of the patch with 10 μM cAMP. The superimposed points are from best fits using a modified Boltzmann equation. Right panel: Dose-response relationship between the voltage shifts of P_o curves against cAMP concentration. Adapted from DiFrancesco (1999) *J. Physiol.* **515**, 367–376 with permission.

HCN channels are blocked by ivabradine and related compounds (Fig. 8.5). The drug works by binding to the channel in its open state and inhibiting the movement of Na^+ (and K^+) through the channel so the rate of diastolic depolarization is slowed and hence heart rate is reduced. Ivabradine is indicated for the symptomatic treatment of chronic stable angina pectoris in patients with normal heart rhythm. It has recently been shown to be effective in the treatment of chronic heart failure, reducing hospitalization and death in this setting (SHIFT trial).

With I_f activation the cells gradually depolarize and the membrane potential begins to reach a voltage range that activates T-type Ca^{2+} channels.

8.4 $I_{Ca,T}$

Activation of T-type Ca^{2+} channels results in an influx of Ca^{2+}, further depolarizing the cells. In Chapter 6 (p. 160) we detailed some of the characteristics of T-type channels but here we explain their role in pacemaker activity. T-type Ca^{2+} channels belong to the LVA class of Ca^{2+} channels that activate at more negative voltages (around –55 mV,

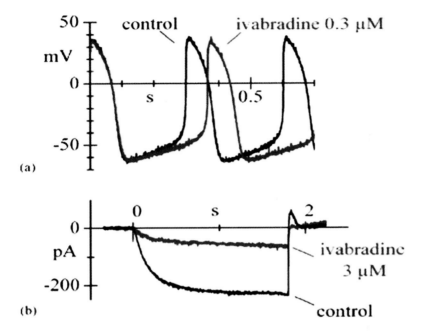

Figure 8.5. Ivabradine inhibition of I_f. Ivabridine reduces the I_f conductance (lower panel, designated (b)), rather than altering the activation curve and therefore decreases the gradient of the diastolic depolarization (upper panel, designated (a)). Reproduced from DiFrancesco (2006) *Pharmacol. Res.* **53**, 399–406 with permission.

reaching a peak around −30 mV) and more rapidly compared with L-type Ca^{2+} channels. Two different isoforms of T-type channels are expressed in the SA node, $Ca_{V3.1}$ (composed of the α1G protein subunit and produced by the CACNA1G gene) and $Ca_{V3.2}$ (comprising α1H and produced by the CACNA1H gene) though some evidence suggests there is more $Ca_{V3.1}$ expressed. The channels have similar electrophysiological properties but can be pharmacologically differentiated on the basis of different sensitivities to Ni^{2+}. Ni^{2+} blocks the $Ca_{V3.2}$ channel with an IC_{50} of about 10–15 μM while $Ca_{V3.1}$ channels are roughly 20 times less sensitive, having an IC_{50} value of about 200–250 μM. Both channels are inhibited by mibefridil. Block of the T-type channels with Ni^{2+} increases the SA node cycle length by about 15% and knocking out the $Ca_{V3.1}$ gene produces a bradycardia. $I_{Ca,T}$ density depends on the species examined, but generally is in the range of 0.5 to 1.0 $A.F^{-1}$. Its reversal potential has not been determined and is assumed to be near the theoretical value predicted using the Nernst equation.

Activation of T-type Ca^{2+} channels occurs as diastolic depolarization reaches their activation range. Ca^{2+} influx depolarizes the cells further and may also trigger localized Ca^{2+} release in the form of Ca^{2+} sparks from the SR. In turn, this local release may stimulate the Na^+/Ca^{2+} exchange and the inward current (produced by Na^+ influx in exchange for Ca^{2+} efflux; see Chapter 5, p. 117) depolarizes the nodal cells further, taking the pacemaker potential towards and beyond the threshold for L-type Ca^{2+} channel activation.

8.5 $I_{Ca,L}$

As we discussed in Chapter 6, $I_{Ca,L}$ activates at potentials more positive than –40 mV and reaches a maximum value around +10 mV. Whereas the current in ventricular myocytes seems to be mainly carried by $Ca_{V1.2}$, the current in the SA node seems to flow mainly through the $Ca_{V1.3}$ isoform. This has a slightly more negative activation potential than $Ca_{V1.2}$, which may allow it to be activated earlier during the diastolic depolarization phase. Activation of this current brings about the slow upstroke of the SA node action potential. The Na^+ channel, $Na_{V1.5}$, which as we have seen is responsible for the fast upstroke of the ventricular action potential, is almost absent from the central SA nodal cells so they rely on Ca^{2+} influx to depolarize fully. More peripheral SA nodal cells appear to express some $Na_{V1.5}$ channels and their existence in these cells would explain their slightly faster upstroke compared with the centrally situated P cells.

8.6 SR Ca^{2+} release in SA nodal cells

Using confocal imaging of Ca^{2+} combined with single-cell voltage clamp of SA nodal cells, Lakatta and colleagues described local, spontaneous Ca^{2+} releases from the SR in the late phase of diastolic depolarization. These local releases appear as 4 to 10 μm wide Ca^{2+} "wavelets" – larger than the aforementioned Ca^{2+} sparks but not propagated like a wave or a much larger event with synchronously released Ca^{2+} – the Ca^{2+} transient. These wavelets appear after the global Ca^{2+} transient has decayed and reach a peak late in the diastolic depolarization phase (Fig. 8.6). Although there is evidence that T-type Ca^{2+} influx promotes their appearance along with Ca^{2+} sparks, voltage clamp studies suggest that many local wavelet occurrences are not affected by inhibition of $I_{Ca,T}$ nor do they require membrane depolarization, rather, most occur spontaneously and rhythmically. The rhythmic and spontaneous Ca^{2+} releases are accompanied by inward current changes with the same periodicity. Lakatta and colleagues therefore developed the view that Ca^{2+}, spontaneously released from the SR into the cytoplasm, is then expelled from the nodal cells by the Na^+/Ca^{2+} exchange which, in so doing, generates an inward current. They propose that this inward current is responsible for accelerating the final (almost exponential) phase of the diastolic depolarization leading to activation of the L-type Ca^{2+} channels, the action potential upstroke and the large, synchronous release of SR Ca^{2+} forming the transient. Thus the rhythmic Ca^{2+} oscillations generate the final part of the depolarization sequence that triggers the SA nodal action potential and has been therefore been termed the "Ca^{2+} clock".

The delay between the depletion of the SR following Ca^{2+} release triggered by the action potential and the appearance of the local Ca^{2+} wavelets during the subsequent diastolic depolarization is the "local Ca^{2+} release period", which Lakatta and colleagues suggest provides the master clock determining the "ticking rate" of the SA node. This period depends greatly on the speed with which the SR is replenished which, in turn, is dependent upon the activity of SERCA. As we discussed in an earlier chapter, SERCA is regulated by PKA- and CaMKII-dependent phosphorylation modulated by β-adrenergic activity and intracellular $[Ca^{2+}]$. Through G-protein coupled signalling pathways, β-adrenergic receptor stimulation increases, and cholinergic receptor stimulation decreases, the basal phosphorylation levels of L- and T-type Ca^{2+} channels and SERCA, leading to an increase and a decrease, respectively, in "ticking rate". A role of the Ca^{2+} clock in pacemaking is controversial in that it is unlikely that it is the single mechanism for

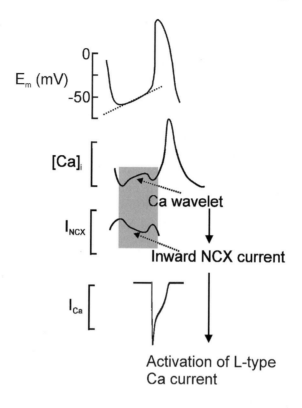

Figure 8.6. During diastolic depolarization (top panel, dotted trace) spontaneous Ca^{2+} release from the SR produces Ca^{2+} wavelets, which are accompanied by inward current changes with the same periodicity probably arising from Na^+/Ca^{2+} exchange expelling the Ca^{2+}. This inward current accelerates the phase of diastolic depolarization leading to activation of the L-type Ca^{2+} channels.

firing and regulating the upstroke timing and speed. It is more likely that the Ca^{2+} clock processes run in parallel with the "membrane clock" that is the net effect of I_f, $I_{Ca,T}$, I_{NaCa} and $I_{Ca,L}$ (and as will be discussed next, I_K). The membrane clock generates and terminates the action potential and initiates the diastolic depolarization, and so guarantees the continual function of the Ca^{2+} clock which, in turn, ensures an appropriately timed upstroke.

8.7 Potassium currents in the SA node

The main potassium currents present in the node are I_{to}, I_{Kr} and I_{Ks}. Their respective roles in repolarizing the cells vary depending on species and the location of the cells within the node (i.e. central P cells or peripheral cells). The initial phase of repolarization is probably achieved by activation of I_{to} because application of 4-aminopyridine prolongs the action potential duration. Similarly, application of E-4031 to block I_{Kr} increases the action potential duration, reduces the maximum diastolic potential and increases cycle length. I_{Kr} activates rapidly in response to depolarization more positive to -40 mV and deactivation of the current contributes to the gradual diastolic depolarization during its early phase. I_{Ks} activates more slowly and does not flow until near the peak of the action potential. Its contribution to repolarization is small under normal conditions but increases during β-adrenergic stimulation.

8.7.1 $I_{K,ACh}$

The existence of acetylcholine-sensitive K^+ channels in SA nodal cells suggests that they are an important mechanism responsible for the slowing of heart rate by vagal stimulation. The binding of acetylcholine to muscarinic M2 receptors activates a G_i-protein, which leads to the activation of K_{ACh} channels. They increase K^+ efflux, hyperpolarizing the cells and stabilizing the membrane potential nearer E_K. In SA nodal cells this slows the rate of diastolic depolarization and therefore heart rate. $I_{K,ACh}$ is carried by a heterotetrameric formation of two monomers of $K_{ir3.1}$ (501 amino acids long) and two of $K_{ir3.4}$ (419 amino acids long). These belong to the inward rectifier family of channels. K_{ACh} channels expressed in the atria are inhibited by membrane stretch so may function as mechano-sensors and provide a mechano-electrical feedback system. A variety of drugs inhibit this channel. Disopyramide, procainamide and pilsicainide block the muscarinic receptors so affecting the activation of the channel, while flecainide and propafenone act as open channel blockers.

However, the idea that K_{ACh} channels were central to the bradycardic effects of vagal stimulation was re-assessed following the observation that ACh was able to inhibit I_f at substantially lower concentrations than $I_{K,ACh}$. This suggested that ACh-induced I_f inhibition, rather than $I_{K,ACh}$ activation is the mechanism underlying the slowing of heart rate.

8.8   Cell heterogeneity

It is important to recognize that the SA node comprises quite a heterogeneous collection of cell sizes and these have very subtle variations in ion channel expression. Therefore, the shape of the action potentials varies among the differing cells. Generally, the small cells in the centre of the node have more negative diastolic membrane potentials and a slower diastolic depolarization phase than the larger peripheral cells, reflecting a lower expression of I_f. The smaller cells also have slower action potential upstrokes, reflecting the lack of Na⁺ channel expression. As the nodal cells spread to the periphery the expression of Na⁺ channels increases and correspondingly their action potentials are faster and the upstroke depolarizations greater.

8.9   Summary

The rhythmical depolarization and repolarization of the pacemaker mechanism can be summarized as follows. I_f is deactivated during the upstroke and the plateau of the SA node action potential. The upstroke is mainly due to $I_{Ca,L}$ though there may be some progressively larger influence of I_{Na} in cells further away from the central area. I_{to} and I_{Kr} are responsible for repolarizing the cells, and as these processes return the membrane potential to more negative voltages (below –40 mV), I_f begins to turn on. The slow activation of inward I_f overcomes the hyperpolarizing outward I_{Kr} and this drives the membrane potential more positive from its maximum diastolic value. With I_f activation the cells gradually depolarize and the membrane potential begins to reach a voltage range that activates T-type Ca^{2+} channels. Ca^{2+} influx and the Ca^{2+} clock-induced activation of I_{NaCa} promote a more rapid depolarization and the upstroke is initiated as L-type Ca^{2+} current is activated.

8.10 Questions

(1) Why do the SA nodal cells have an unstable membrane potential?

(2) What is the unusual characteristic of I_f and describe why this current plays a role in pacemaking?

(3) Discuss the effects of the neurotransmitters, noradrenaline and ACh on I_f.

(4) Describe the "Ca clock" hypothesis of pacemaking.

8.11 Bibliography

8.11.1 *Reviews*

DiFrancesco, D. (2006). Funny channels in the control of cardiac rhythm and mode of action of selective blockers. *Pharmacol. Res.* **53**, 399–406.

Maltsev, V.A. and Lakatta, E.G. (2008). Dynamic interactions of an intracellular Ca^{2+} clock and membrane ion channel clock underlie robust initiation and regulation of cardiac pacemaker function. *Cardiovasc. Res.* **77**, 274–284.

Ono, K., and Iijima, T. (2010). Cardiac T-type Ca^{2+} channels in the heart. *J. Mol. Cell. Cardiol.* **48**, 65–70.

Yamada, M., Inanobe, A. and Kurachi, Y. (1998). G-Protein regulation of potassium ion channels. *Pharmacol. Rev.* **50**, 723–757.

8.11.2 *Original papers*

Brown, H.F., DiFrancesco, D. and Noble, S.J. (1979). How does adrenaline accelerate the heart? *Nature* **280**, 235–236.

Bohm, M., Swedberg, K., Komajda, M. *et al.* (2010). Heart rate as a risk factor in chronic heart failure (SHIFT): the association between heart rate and outcomes in a randomised placebo-controlled trial. *Lancet* **376**, 886–894.

DiFrancesco, D. (1991). The contribution of the "pacemaker current" (i$_f$) to generation of spontaneous activity in rabbit sino-atrial node myocytes. *J. Physiol.* **434**, 23–40.

DiFrancesco, D. (1999). Dual allosteric modulation of pacemaker (f) channels by cAMP and voltage in rabbit SA node. *J. Physiol.* **515**, 367–376.

Noma, A. and Irisawa, H. (1976). Membrane currents in the rabbit sinoatrial node cell as studied by the double microelectrode method. *Pflugers Arch.* **364**, 45–52.

Vinogradova, T.M., Brochet, D.X.P., Sirenko, S. *et al.* (2010). Sarcoplasmic reticulum Ca^{2+} pumping kinetics regulates timing of local Ca^{2+} releases and spontaneous beating rate of rabbit sinoatrial node pacemaker cells. *Circ. Res.* **107**, 767–775.

Chapter 9

Conduction, Arrhythmias and
Anti-arrhythmic Agents

In this chapter we are going to examine the way one action potential in a
cell excites a neighbouring cell leading to the propagation of the
excitatory impulse throughout the heart and then how this mechanism
can be disturbed causing arrhythmias. Finally, we will examine how anti-
arrhythmic medication works to restore normal cardiac rhythm and rate
and prevent the formation of dangerous arrhythmias.

9.1 Chapter objectives

After reading this chapter you should be able to:

- Understand how excitation propagates from cell to cell
- Describe different ways impulse propagation can be disturbed
- Describe the different ways impulse generation can be altered
- Understand the basic mechanisms that underlie the action of
  anti-arrhythmic drug intervention

9.2 Simple conduction

A very simplified model of cardiac impulse propagation is one where
there is a single line of cells attached to each other at intercalated discs
within which lie gap junctions. Using this model the mechanism
underlying propagation can be split in a series of simple steps (Fig. 9.1).

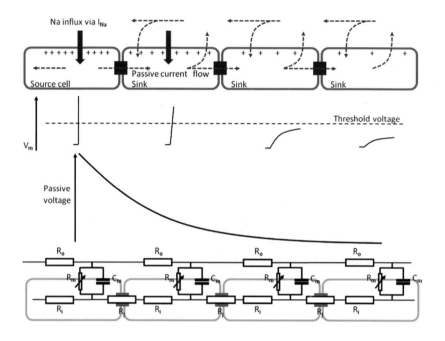

Figure 9.1. Conduction in a single strand of ventricular myocytes. Na$^+$ influx occurs in the cell at the left producing a rapid upstroke and a depolarization of the membrane potential (V_m). The inside of the cell becomes positive. A small current flows from this point source to the neighbouring cells (-----►) which are sinks of current. The flow depends on the resistances of the cytoplasm (R_i) and the gap junctions (R_j). This flow of current results in a passive axial decay of voltage along the strand. The completed electrical circuit is formed by a corresponding current flowing through the extracellular fluid with resistance R_o. The local current flow sets up local membrane potential changes which are not propagated but decay exponentially. If the active cell depolarizes its neighbouring cell sufficiently for it to reach its threshold potential then an action potential will be generated in the neighbouring cell. If threshold is not reached then insufficient Na$^+$ channels will be activated and an action potential will not be evoked and propagation will cease. The passive voltage decays exponentially along the axis of the strand. The equivalent electrical circuit is illustrated in the lowest part of the figure. This is similar to the electrical models used to calculate the flow of electric current and the corresponding voltage changes along passive (i.e. not firing) neurones. This passive current spread could be closely modelled by mathematical descriptions of electrical signal decay in telegraph cables originally developed by Lord Kelvin and colleagues in the 1850s (so-called cable theory).

Firstly, an action potential has been generated in the cell on the leftmost part of the strand. As we have established in earlier chapters, a local change in ionic conductance produces an influx of Na^+ into the cell which causes it to depolarize, and the charge across its surface membrane changes from being normally negative on the inside to being positive (with respect to the extracellular solution). The change in membrane potential is initially localized to the cell but a small current will flow between it and its neighbouring cells that have different polarity. This local circuit current is produced by positive charge passing from the active (depolarized) cell to the resting cells and spreading axially along the strand of cells, becoming exponentially smaller as it does so. The completed electrical circuit is formed by a corresponding current flowing in the extracellular fluid.

Secondly, if large enough, this current will depolarize its neighbouring, resting cell serving as a source of electrical charge while the resting cell, together with other resting cells, constitutes an electrical sink. If the active cell provides sufficient charge to its neighbouring resting cell for it to depolarize enough to reach its threshold potential then an action potential will be generated in that neighbouring cell. The newly excited cell then changes from being a sink to being a new current source for the cells further down the strand and so the action potential (and the wave of depolarization) propagates from one cell to the next. The size of the source current is largely controlled by the size of I_{Na} and $I_{Ca,L}$ in comparison to the early repolarizing currents, I_{to} and I_{Kur}.

It is important to note that the key factor in this chain of events is the local current flow from a depolarized cell to its resting neighbours. The local current flow sets up local membrane potential changes that are not propagated but decay exponentially. As long as this *electrotonic* spread of potential remains sufficiently large that it triggers an action potential in the next cell, then propagation will continue. The main factor governing the spread of local current flow is the intracellular resistance (R_i).

R_m is the membrane resistance, a variable quantity that determines how much the membrane potential will change in response to a current flowing across the membrane. It depends on the number of open channels and the size of the cell.

The greater this value then the less will be the spread of electrotonic current. The distance of current spread and therefore voltage change along the cells in the strand is expressed in terms of a length constant (λ):

$$\lambda = \sqrt{\frac{R_m}{R_i}} \tag{9.1}$$

λ in cardiac tissue is about 2 mm.

The positively induced voltage at a point (x) along the strand from its maximum point (V_o) where current density is greatest is defined by the following equation:

$$V_x = V_0 e^{-\frac{x}{\lambda}} \tag{9.2}$$

This means that at a distance (λ) along the strand, the voltage will have decreased to 37% of its maximum value (Fig. 9.2).

R_i becomes smaller as cell diameter increases and its value along the strand depends upon the number and type of gap junctions that connect the cells. Gap junctions are specialized intercellular connections that provide low resistance pathways between cells (Fig. 9.3). One gap junction comprises two connexons (also called hemichannels), each embedded in the surface membranes of apposing cells, which dock together across the intercellular space or gap to form a channel that allows various ions and molecules up to 1 kDa in size to pass freely between the two cells. Each connexon consists of six individual connexin proteins, so a fully formed gap junction is a dodecamer of connexins. Connexins have various isoforms with the main differences occurring in

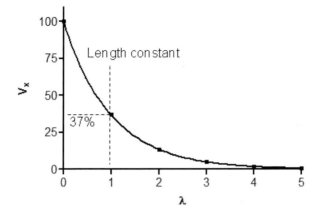

Figure 9.2.   The decay of voltage along a strand of cells.

the carboxyl tail, which is the region involved in the regulation of channel properties. In the heart the main connexin (Cx) types are 40, 43 and 45. These vary in their degree of expression and in the way they combine to form gap junctions throughout various parts of the heart, with compatibility determined by the amino acid sequence of the second extracellular loop, as well as by specific intracellular domains. Ventricular myocytes mainly express Cx43 with small quantities of Cx45, while atrial myocytes express Cx40 and Cx43 with some Cx45. Myocytes forming the conduction system chiefly express Cx40 and Cx45. It is thought that these variations contribute to the differences in propagation speed observed in different parts of the heart. The gap junction conductance between cells appears to be about the same as the cytoplasmic conductance of the cells, so that the time taken by the wave of depolarization to cross the gap junction (approximately 0.1 ms) is about the same as it takes to traverse the length of the cell. The high level of gap junction expression is why heart tissue is considered to behave as a functional syncytium of cells: an action potential generated in one region will spread rapidly and efficiently to others so that there is coordinated contraction of the chambers.

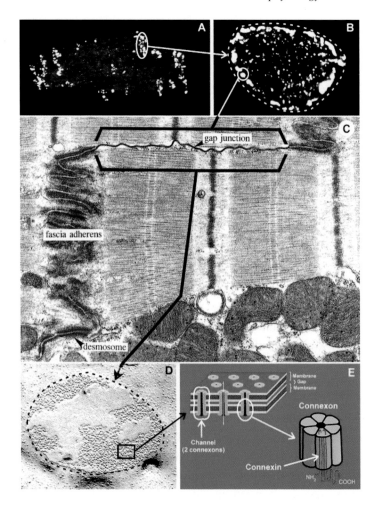

Figure 9.3. Gap junction organization and structure. Panel A: Clusters of gap junctions in ventricular myocytes at the intercalated discs revealed with Cx43 immunostaining. Panel B: Clusters of gap junctions at one intercalated disc viewed face-on. One of these areas (circled) corresponds to a single gap junction, as seen by electron microscopy in Panels C and D. Panel C: Thin-section electron micrograph illustrating the three types of cell junction of the intercalated disc. Gap junctions have formed where the adjacent plasma membrane profiles run in close contact, separated by a gap of 2 nm. The fascia adherens and the desmosome are characterized by a much wider intermembrane space (25 nm). Panel D: Viewing the membrane *en face* by freeze-fracture reveals the gap junction as a cluster of particles (connexons). Panel E: Each gap junction channel consists of two connexons and each connexon of six connexins. From Severs (2000) *BioEssays* **22**, 188–199 with permission.

Changes in R_i or inward depolarizing current flow affect, independently, the propagation velocity. Propagation velocity is proportional to the square root of the maximal upstroke (phase 0) velocity (dV_m/dt) and inversely proportional to the square root of R_i. The fastest propagation is found in Purkinje fibres (approximately 2 m.s^{-1}) and the slowest occurs in ventricular muscle (approximately 0.5 m.s^{-1}).

The initial action potential generation could propagate in either direction along the strand. Normally, it does not do so because the region just behind the wave of depolarization will be refractory and so forward (in the above example left to right) conduction is easier to maintain.

The success of propagation depends on a quantity that is related to the source–sink relationship called the safety factor (SF). SF is defined as the ratio of charge generated (by the source cell) to charge consumed (by the sink cell or cells). A value greater than 1 indicates that more charge is produced during excitation than is needed to cause the onward downstream excitation of the sink cell so successful propagation ensues. However, suppose there is a decrease in the density of functional sodium channels due to say partial and local pharmacological blockade. In this area of tissue less source current can be produced so reducing its excitability. This affects both conduction velocity (because it depends on the square root of the upstroke velocity) and the SF for propagation. If excitability decreases to the point when the SF falls below 1, then conduction between one cell and the next cannot continue and impulse propagation ceases.

We have examined a very simple case of wave-front propagation in one dimension. Propagation in two dimensions is more complex because most cells are coupled to several others in the transverse as well as in the longitudinal direction. Cardiac tissue has the property of anisotropy whereby the conduction velocity (CV) is much greater longitudinally compared with transversely because the cells are much more electrically coupled in the former direction, due to most gap junctions being located at the ends of cells. The degree of anisotropy is defined by the anisotropy ratio (AR). $AR = CV_{long}/CV_{trans}$ and the main factors affecting this ratio

Conduction pathway

Action potentials generated by the SA node (detailed in Chapter 8) spread throughout the right and left atria triggering their contraction. The atria are electrically insulated from the ventricles by a "fibrous skeleton" formed from dense connective tissue. This insulating layer not only electrically separates the atria and ventricles, but also anchors the heart valves by forming supportive ring structures at the attachment points of the valves. The fibrous skeleton is broken usually at one point by the bundle of His, which forms a conduction pathway through it made by spindle-shaped myocytes. The structure is named after Wilhelm His, who discovered it in 1893. Just superior to the bundle of His lies the atrioventricular (AV) node situated on the right atrial side of the fibrous skeleton near the ostium of the coronary sinus. It is difficult to determine the point when the AV node ends and the His bundle begins because there is a gradual transition in cell morphology from one area to the other. The AV node is composed of myocytes with few intercalated discs so the junctional resistance between nodal cells is increased compared with ventricular tissue. This feature increases the impulse conduction time through the node (CV = 0.05 m.s^{-1}) so allowing sufficient time for atrial systole before the ventricles are activated. Other electrical connections between the atria and ventricles sometimes exist and these form "accessory pathways" that can cause arrhythmias. The His bundle divides near the top of the ventricular septum into the left and right bundle branches. These run along each side of the septum carrying the impulse towards the apex of the heart. The bundle branches conduct the impulses at a very rapid velocity (about 2 m.s^{-1}) because they are insulated from the ventricular myocardium by a connective tissue sheath. The bundle branches divide into an extensive sub-endocardial network of Purkinje fibres discovered in 1839 by Jan Purkyně. They are larger than ventricular myocytes, but have fewer myofibrils and consequently are weakly contractile. They are specialized conducting fibres, which extend well into the ventricular myocardium. They appear to have a sheath of connective tissue surrounding them until they meet ventricular myocytes. The insulating sheath helps maintain a fast conduction velocity and prevents the lateral spread of conduction. Rapid conduction, Purkinje fibre pathway and emergence ensure an even spread of depolarization from the inner (endocardium) to the outer (epicardium) ventricular walls and from apex to base of the whole heart.

are cell geometry and the sizes and distribution of gap junctions. The highest AR is found in the crista terminalis, the smooth muscular ridge in the superior portion of right atrium (AR ≈ 10) and the lowest in the ventricles (AR ≈ 2). These anisotropic ratios are consistent with function because the crista terminalis provides highly directed propagation from the SA node to the right atrium, while in the ventricle most of the impulse conduction is carried and distributed by the Purkinje fibres with inter-myocyte conduction playing a smaller role.

When the impulse leaves the Purkinje network there is an elliptical rather than a circular spread of membrane depolarization away from the point source of current. Due to the low anisotropy of the working ventricular myocardium, wave-fronts tend to spread and not travel in straight lines. Wave-fronts may encounter either functional (areas of temporarily unexcitable tissue) or structural obstacles (areas of dead or non-excitable tissue) and these cause the wave-front to deviate, turn and become curved. The radius of curvature of the wave-front can also determine the propagation velocity. Below a critical value of radius, conduction can start to fail because the wave-front rotates into an area that is refractory.

9.3 Arrhythmias

Arrhythmias are due to disturbances in either impulse generation or impulse propagation. They can be broadly classified into bradyarrhythmias, in which the heart beats at an unusually slow rate and so, in the absence of any increase in stroke volume, may result in low cardiac output, and tachyarrhythmias, in which the heart may contract too quickly to fill the ventricles adequately with blood with a similar result of low cardiac output.

9.3.1 *Disturbances in impulse generation*

Disturbances in generation arise from areas of the heart initiating impulses independently from the normal generating site, the SA node. This phenomenon is termed automaticity and any area of the heart that initiates such impulses is termed an ectopic focus. Ectopic foci can cause additional beats or take over (capture) the normal pacemaker impulses. The foci result from hypoxic or ischaemic insults to the tissue, sympathetic overstimulation, enlargement of (particularly atrial) cells, slowing of the normal intrinsic heart rate, electrolyte disturbances and drug actions. Many of these stimuli for foci production cause triggered arrhythmias. Triggered arrhythmias are due to extra action potentials being produced as a result of spontaneous depolarizations that reach a threshold for Na^+ or Ca^{2+} channel activation. The spontaneous depolarizations can form either during the repolarization phases of the action potentials or during the diastolic (phase 4) periods. The former type is called an early afterdepolarization (EAD) and the latter, a delayed afterdepolarization (DAD). Both types of afterdepolarization may play a role in the generation of ventricular arrhythmias and both are believed to be the result of abnormalities of intracellular calcium handling although the mechanisms responsible for their initiation are different.

9.3.1.1 *Early afterdepolarization (EAD)*

EADs tend to occur when several key situations prevail: the action potential is prolonged, there is bradycardia and there is a reduction in outward, repolarizing current. Examples of the last situation may be as a consequence of hypokalaemia and a resultant decrease in I_{K1}, or congenital channel defects producing long QT syndrome. As repolarization proceeds in these settings, any abnormal increase in net inward current may overcome the repolarization process causing a small depolarization. EADs usually occur near the end of the plateaux of action potentials in a voltage range roughly between +10 mV and –20 mV. As we discussed in Chapter 6 (p. 152), $I_{Ca,L}$ activates within this range of voltages and measurements of the current show a significant region of overlap between the activation and inactivation versus voltage relationships, giving rise to a so-called "window" (Fig. 9.4). What this means is that as the action potential repolarizes into this range of voltages, a proportion of $I_{Ca,L}$ can activate or reactivate. If this current is large enough to overcome the repolarization process, a significant depolarization will occur that can result in triggering of more SR Ca^{2+} release and an aftercontraction (Fig. 9.4). The triggered SR Ca^{2+} release

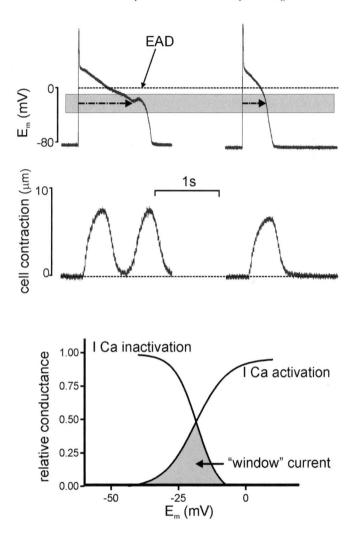

Figure 9.4. The top traces show action potentials recorded from the same cell. The prolonged action potential (left) has induced an EAD by reactivating some $I_{Ca,L}$, which has triggered an aftercontraction seen on the trace below. $I_{Ca,L}$ activation and inactivation show a significant region of overlap (lower graph) producing "window" current. The voltage range of the window current is shaded in the panel with the action potential traces. When the action potential duration is shorter (right) (shown by the arrow), the repolarization process overcomes any reactivation of $I_{Ca,L}$.

causes more inward current mediated by I_{NCX} and this adds to the formation of the EAD. This type of afterdepolarization can initiate a form of ventricular tachycardia called torsades de pointes. While $I_{Ca,L}$ reactivation may be the main mechanism involved in EAD production, it is now more accepted that poor regulation of cytoplasmic [Ca^{2+}] may also contribute. This is because the cytoplasmic (or more specifically the sub-sarcolemmal) [Ca^{2+}] determines the size of the I_{NCX} which may, depending on circumstances, provide enough depolarizing current to induce reactivation of $I_{Ca,L}$ or evoke an EAD itself.

9.3.1.2 *Delayed afterdepolarization (DAD)*

DADs are most frequently observed under conditions in which cytoplasmic [Ca^{2+}] and SR Ca^{2+} content are increased. These situations often occur when heart rates are high or in the presence of β-receptor agonists or cardiotonic steroids. DADs take place during the diastolic interval and are quite distinct from any membrane potential changes associated with the action potential. They are caused by activation of Ca^{2+}-dependent currents following spontaneous releases of Ca^{2+} from the SR. The release of Ca^{2+} into the cytoplasm activates the Na^{+}/Ca^{2+} exchange and, in some species, Ca^{2+}-activated Cl^{-} current ($I_{Cl,Ca}$). The release of Ca^{2+} often causes an aftercontraction and the inward currents depolarize the cell. If the depolarizations are large enough they may reach a voltage range that will start to activate Na^{+} channels and a premature upstroke may ensue.

9.3.2 *Disturbances in impulse propagation*

Disruptions to impulse propagation or conduction generally fall into one of two categories; blocks in the excitation pathways or re-entrant excitation. Blocks in the excitation pathways tend to occur either in the fast conducting bundle of specialized heart cells that branch along the interventricular septum to convey excitation to the right and left ventricles, or at or near the AV node which impairs propagation from the atria to the ventricles. Re-entrant excitation can occur locally in a small region of any area of the heart or can affect the organ more globally and involve upper and lower chambers. Re-entry will only happen if two conditions prevail. Firstly, there needs to be some cardiac tissue which only allows conduction in one direction, i.e. exhibits so-called unidirectional block. Secondly, the speed of conduction through the unidirectional area must be slow enough that tissue is no longer refractory when the impulse reaches the distal side of the area (Fig. 9.5).

9.3.2.1 *Bundle branch block*

In bundle branch block the wave of depolarization travels from the SA node via the atria to the interventricular septum normally so the PR interval of the ECG is normal. The ventricles are still stimulated by regular sinus node function. However, if there is abnormal conduction through either the right or left bundle branches there will be a delay in excitation to some parts of the ventricles so the normal excitation sequence will be longer. The extra time taken for depolarization of the left and/or right ventricles causes a widening of the QRS complex (so it becomes longer than 0.12 s). The causes of bundle branch block are mainly aortic stenosis, coronary artery disease and myocardial infarction, and the condition is associated with impaired left ventricular function.

Torsades de pointes

Torsades de pointes is a French expression meaning "twisting of the points". It is a form of ventricular tachycardia that produces a characteristic ECG in which the QRS complex "twists" around the isoelectric baseline. It is often initiated by an EAD forming as a result of the prolongation of the action potential. The EAD produces a shorter than normal extra action potential and an aftercontraction. The extrasystolic event appears as an R on T wave disturbance on the ECG. This extra systole is followed by a compensatory pause to allow more chamber filling and the following beat is larger, not only because of Starling's law, but also the SR has had time to fill more completely. The larger contraction and the longer than normal action potential can together produce large repolarization and electromechanical gradients across the myocardial wall and re-entry events can start to occur. If these continue, a circular pattern of ventricular depolarization takes place resulting in QRS complexes that continuously vary in their axes around the isoelectric baseline. Torsades de pointes is associated with a fall in arterial blood pressure and syncope and can degenerate into ventricular fibrillation.

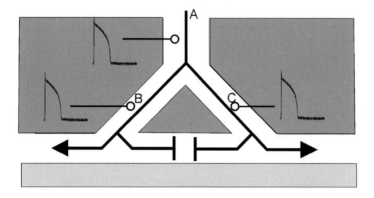

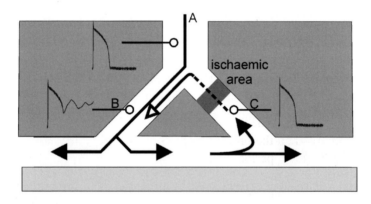

Figure 9.5. The phenomenon of re-entry. Upper panel: Excitation proceeds down branch A where it divides and travels along branches B and C. Electrodes placed at these points record normal action potentials. When excitatory wave-fronts meet they cancel each other. Lower panel: An area of tissue becomes damaged causing gap junction redistribution and cell depolarization (dark shading) so that it is only capable of conducting in one direction. The wave of excitation travels past electrode B and splits as before. There is no corresponding wave advancing towards C because of the area of block. The excitation wave moves anti-clockwise towards electrode C from B. The wave-front then moves through the unidirectional block (dark shading) backwards (retrograde) with reduced velocity. When it reaches the tissue through which the previous impulses have travelled, the tissue has recovered from its refractory period and is now excitable again. The wave of excitation will then re-enter this branch, pass electrode B a second time depolarizing the tissue much earlier than normal, and a circular pathway is initiated.

9.3.2.2 *Re-entry*

Re-entry phenomena are usually described as follows. In Fig. 9.5 the cardiac tissue could be any branching network (ventricular muscle or Purkinje fibre). Excitation would proceed normally down the main branch (A) where it would divide and travel down branches B and C. Electrodes placed at these points record the waves of excitation. If the branched pathways meet more distally the action potentials would cancel each other due to refractory conditions being set up.

Suppose that an area of tissue becomes hypoxic such that it is only capable of conducting in one direction. This could arise because of gap junction redistribution and cell depolarization. The wave of excitation travels past electrode B and splits as before. This time there is no corresponding wave advancing towards C because of the unidirectional block in the shaded area. An action potential is recorded at electrode C but this is produced by the excitation wave moving backwards (retrograde) towards it. This wave-front moves through the unidirectional block (shaded area) but does so slowly because conduction velocity is reduced in this area. When the excitatory wave moves past the block, the tissue through which the previous impulses have travelled has recovered from its refractory period and is now excitable again. The action potentials will then re-enter this branch, pass electrode B a second time depolarizing the tissue much earlier than normal and a circular pathway of now much higher frequency impulses is initiated. The process of re-entry is therefore very dependent on a unidirectionally conducting area of tissue and the time of arrival of the slowed and re-entering impulse.

If the excitation impulse traverses the area with block too quickly, the next area of tissue may not be excitable because it may still be refractory. It will then not be able to conduct and the wave-front will be extinguished. Sites of re-entry may only affect a small area of tissue but could become large to affect whole chambers if conditions – timing and refractory state – are right.

Following myocardial infarction, the affected parts of the heart will comprise areas of relatively normal myocardium connected to regions with reduced intercellular coupling or necrotic tissue which impose structural non-uniformities. It is easy to understand that this substrate could cause changes in excitability, conduction and the spread of depolarizing current and so provides a setting that makes re-entrant arrhythmias more likely.

9.4 Anti-arrhythmics

The purpose of using anti-arrhythmic medication is to restore normal cardiac rhythm and rate and prevent the formation of dangerous arrhythmias. There are several ways these goals can be achieved:

(1) Altering the conduction velocity
(2) Altering cell excitability by changing the duration of the ERP
(3) Suppressing abnormal automaticity

9.4.1 *Inhibiting Na$^+$ channels*

Drugs that block Na$^+$ channels will decrease the speed at which the cells depolarize and therefore will reduce the conduction velocity. Some Na$^+$ channel blockers will also increase the action potential duration and these will therefore increase the refractory period and so decrease the likelihood of re-entry occurring. As a result they are useful drugs for treating tachyarrhythmias caused by re-entry. Vaughan Williams classified these substances in one group (see Table 9.1) because they generally decreased the speed of the phase 0 upstroke and therefore conduction velocity. Subsequently they have been sub-classified on the basis of their effects not only on conduction velocity, but also on the ECG and action potential duration – therefore refractory period – and the speed in onset of use-dependent block of the Na$^+$ channel.

The Na$^+$ channel blockers generally bind to the *inactivated* Na$^+$ channel from the intracellular side. The channels are pushed into their inactivated state by depolarization and so repetitive shifts to more depolarized potentials by trains of stimuli promote binding of more drug molecules to the channels. This explains why these compounds are "use

Class	Channel block	ECG changes	APD	Speed of block	Examples
1A	intermediate	PR and QT prolongation	increase	intermediate	quinidine, procainamide, disopyramide
1B	weak	no change	small decrease	rapid	lidocaine, tocainide, mexiletine
1C	strong	QRS prolongation	no change	slow	flecainide, propafenone, moracizine

Table 9.1. Vaughan Williams Class 1 drugs.

dependent" i.e. their block increases with channel activity. The drugs bind to the S6 regions of domains III and IV. The exact sites are not known but are influenced by point mutations to the P loop. Although these drugs also affect the Na^+ channels in the nervous system and are generally classified as local anaesthetics, there is reason to believe the cardiac isoforms of the channels may have different affinities for binding these drugs (e.g. the relative insensitivity of $Na_{V1.5}$ to TTX compared with other isoforms). Their profound effects on the heart are probably a result of the prolonged action potential in the tissue compared with neurones. Cardiac cells spend a longer time in the depolarized state and this seems to determine the degree of channel block. This effect is also observed within cardiac cell types. Local anaesthetics affect ventricular cells more than atrial cells with the former having longer action potential durations.

These drugs have similar chemical structures yet the mechanisms of their block are slightly different. They all show use-dependent block, but lidocaine has a higher affinity for inactivated channels in comparison with those in a closed state. Flecainide appears to block Na^+ channels following their opening (so-called open channel block). It is probable

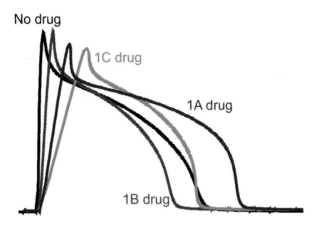

Figure 9.6. Action potential changes with various Class 1 drugs.

that the differences in pK_a of the molecules (and hence their charge at physiological pH) rather than their structure determines their mechanism of block.

The aim in using the Class 1 anti-arrhythmic agents is to improve cardiac function by restoring sinus rhythm and so controlling ventricular rate. The drugs slow the upstroke of the action potential and therefore slow conduction and increase the threshold for excitation of the cells (Fig. 9.6). The class 1A drugs increase APD and therefore the effective refractory period is increased. The drugs are used to treat supraventricular and ventricular tachycardias because they slow impulse propagation across the atria and through the AV node. The class 1A drugs, which prolong the refractory period, also help decrease the likelihood of automaticity and re-entry occurring.

9.4.2 *Inhibiting Ca^{2+} channels*

Calcium channel blockers mainly affect impulse initiation at the SA node (see Chapter 8) and reduce conduction through the AV node. They also decrease cardiac contractility (i.e. they have a negative inotropic effect) and dilate the coronary arteries, which increases myocardial oxygen supply.

Verapamil (a phenylalkylamine) and diltiazem (a benzothiazepine) are used as anti-arrhythmics in preference to the dihypropyridines (e.g. nifedipine, nitrendipine) since the latter group act more preferentially on smooth muscle cells where they lead to vasodilation; a key feature for anti-hypertensive therapies. These compounds have little anti-arrhythmic action. Verapamil and diltiazem are Vaughan Williams class IV anti-arrhythmics. They bind to both L- and T-type Ca^{2+} channels that, in the nodal cells, govern the upstroke of the action potential and the slope of the pacemaker potentials respectively. They generally have no effect on APD in these cells but slow the upstroke and decrease the slope of the pacemaker potential, so reducing the firing rate of abnormal pacemaker sites within the heart and the velocity of impulse conduction at the AV node. This helps block sites of spontaneous pacemaker activity and re-entry that can cause supraventricular tachyarrhythmias such as atrial fibrillation, atrial flutter and paroxysmal supraventricular tachycardia. Any abnormal automaticity dependent on Ca^{2+} channels will be reduced by their action so they will stop triggered activity due to EADs (which depend on Ca^{2+} channel re-opening during the later part of the plateau) and DADs (which result from Ca^{2+} overload of the cell).

Available evidence suggests that the binding sites for the Ca^{2+} channel antagonists are on the S6 trans-membrane segment of domains III and IV close to the selectivity filter of the α-subunit which, when occupied, change its gating behaviour. The different classes of drug bind to separate, but allosterically linked sites. They reduce the whole cell I_{Ca} without changing the size of the single-channel current. This occurs because the drug binding causes a negative shift in the voltage dependence of inactivation of the channel which, in turn, decreases channel availability and reduces the probability of channel opening. Diltiazem can block the channels from either the outside or inside of the cells but verapamil blocks from the cytoplasmic side. Binding is increased by depolarization and decreased by hyperpolarization and block can occur to both activated and inactivated forms of the channels.

Channels become progressively more inhibited with repetitive depolarization indicating that the Ca^{2+} channel blockers are also use dependent.

9.4.3 *Inhibiting K^+ channels*

The rationale for using K^+ channel blockers is to delay repolarization (phase 3) so increasing cell action potential duration and effective refractory period. This group of drugs belong to class III of the Vaughan Williams categorization and all increase cellular APD and the Q-T interval of the ECG. On the one hand prolonging the effective refractory period is useful for decreasing re-entry, but on the other, doing so can be pro-arrhythmic because the prolongation can lead to the formation of EADs that can trigger torsades de pointes ventricular arrhythmias. There are some well-established Class III agents, e.g. amiodarone and sotolol. Amiodarone has an extremely complex mechanism of action and for a full explanation the reader is referred to the review by Kodama *et al.* (1997). The drug prolongs the APD by binding to some types of K^+ channel and so slows repolarization, but it also blocks Na^+ and Ca^{2+} channels as well as α- and β-adrenoceptors. Additionally, it may bring about some subtle anti-arrhythmic remodelling of cells probably through a modulation of gene expression of ion channels. It rarely causes torsades de pointes but can produce severe side effects, in particular thyroid dysfunction and lung fibrosis.

Sotalol is a non-specific β-adrenergic receptor blocker that has K^+ channel blocking properties. Its most serious side effect is torsades de pointes because of the profound QT prolongation.

Class III drugs such as sotalol and amiodarone not only block K^+ channels but also have a variety of other properties. The newer class III agents such as dofetilide and E-4031 were developed to have more specific K^+ channel blocking activity. Dofetilide selectively blocks I_{Kr} in a voltage-dependent manner. Block is greater at more depolarized potentials. Of clinical importance is that the block of I_{Kr} becomes progressively greater as the extracellular K^+ concentration is reduced, because any patient with hypokalaemia would suffer a disproportionately increased action potential duration with pro-arrhythmic consequences.

9.4.4 *Class II anti-arrhythmics*

The Vaughan Williams classification puts β-blockers in this category. The rationale for their use as anti-arrhythmics is that these compounds will block β_1-adrenergic receptors and decrease sympathetic activity. Blockade of the β_1-adrenoreceptor reduces $G_{\alpha s}$-mediated activation of adenylate cyclase and decreases production of cAMP. This will decrease sinus node activity so heart rate slows. Conduction through the AV node also slows because $I_{Ca,L}$ will be reduced. This decrease in conduction velocity prevents global re-entry. Ectopic foci will also tend to be reduced because β_1-adrenergic blockade will slow any diastolic depolarization that may precede such occurrences. These drugs therefore form an important part of an evolving therapeutic regime for patients with atrial fibrillation.

9.4.5 *Other drugs*

9.4.5.1 *Adenosine*

In the heart, adenosine binds to a type 1 (also called A1) G-protein coupled receptor activating a pertussis toxin-sensitive pathway. Activation of this pathway opens ATP- and ACh-sensitive K^+ channels, which hyperpolarize the cells. The mechanisms that bring about the G-protein activation of these channels are different. The $G_{\beta \delta}$ subunit combination binds to regions of the K_{ACh} channel causing its activation and the G_α subunit activates K_{ATP} channels. Activation of these K^+ channels tends to reduce the gradient of diastolic depolarization in SA nodal cells, therefore decreases heart rate and slows the generation of the upstroke at the AV node reducing atrial to ventricular conduction velocity. It is therefore used in the treatment of supraventricular tachycardias because by reducing atrial to ventricular conduction velocity the AV nodal area has a longer ERP, which inhibits re-entry. Adenosine is often administered intravenously. It activates K_{ATP} channels leading to smooth muscle hyperpolarization and vascular relaxation. It exerts a direct depressant effect on the SA node when administered, which can be sufficient to cause asystole for a few seconds. The heart rate then transiently increases due to baroreceptor reflexes responding to systemic hypotension.

9.4.5.2 *Digoxin*

Digoxin is a cardiac glycoside extracted from the foxglove plant. We discussed its cellular mechanism of action in Chapter 5 (pp. 122–123). It is a positive inotrope most often used in the treatment of atrial fibrillation or atrial flutter, particularly when the sufferer also has congestive heart failure. Whether it can be classed as a true anti-arrhythmic is debatable.

It has two mechanisms of action. It inhibits the Na^+/K^+ ATPase so increasing intracellular $[Na^+]$ and subsequently shifting the equilibrium potential of the Na^+/Ca^{2+} exchange. This shift reduces the beat-to-beat efflux of Ca^{2+} from the cells and a new steady-state balance at a higher level of intracellular $[Ca^{2+}]$ is achieved. Digoxin therefore increases the strength of contraction and so improves the pumping function of the heart. At first sight this improvement would seem very beneficial and, indeed, the drug used to be a standard treatment for the failing heart. However, it has a very narrow therapeutic "window" and so toxic effects of the drug are common. Crucially, it did not demonstrate any mortality benefit in patients with congestive heart failure so its use has declined. It is still very valuable for patients with atrial fibrillation and coexistent heart failure and in those with normal sinus rhythm but who have impaired left ventricular systolic function, which has not improved with diuretics and ACE inhibitors. The downside of improving contractility by increasing stored Ca^{2+} is that automaticity can be increased. However, increased intracellular $[Ca^{2+}]$ probably activates outward currents, which will lengthen phase 4 and in the SA node will lead to a decrease in heart rate.

Digoxin's second mode of action is as a parasympathomimetic. For reasons poorly understood it increases vagal activity to the heart so slowing the firing of the SA node. In the AV node this effect slows conduction and ventricular excitation, which is useful in the treatment of patients with atrial fibrillation.

9.5 Summary

- Excitation of a cell at one end of strand of single cells causes a small current to flow from this point source to the neighbouring cells which are sinks of current. The current flow depends on the cytoplasmic and gap junctional resistances and results in a passive decay of voltage along the strand which is not propagated. If the active cell depolarizes its neighbouring cell sufficiently for it to reach its threshold potential then an action potential will be generated in that cell. If threshold is not reached then insufficient Na^+ channels will be activated, an action potential will not be evoked and propagation will cease.
- The main factor governing the spread of local current flow is the intracellular resistance (R_i). The greater this value then the less will be the spread of electrotonic current. The distance of current spread and therefore voltage change along the cells in the strand is expressed in terms of a length constant (λ). R_i becomes smaller as cell diameter increases and its value along a strand of cells depends upon the number and type of gap junctions that connect neighbouring cells.
- Gap junctions are specialized intercellular connections that provide low resistance pathways between cells. Clusters of gap junctions form at intercalated discs and where the plasma membrane of the adjacent cell runs in close contact. Each gap junction is formed from a cluster of connexons with each channel consisting of two connexons and each connexon of six connexins.
- Cardiac tissue has the property of anisotropy whereby the CV is much greater longitudinally compared with transversely. Cells are more electrically coupled longitudinally because most gap junctions are located at the ends of cells. The degree of anisotropy is defined by the anisotropy ratio (AR). AR =

CV_{long}/CV_{trans} and the main factors affecting this ratio are cell geometry and the sizes and distribution of gap junctions.

- Arrhythmias are due to disturbances in either impulse generation or impulse propagation. They can be broadly classified into bradyarrhythmias and tachyarrhythmias.

- EADs tend to occur when several situations prevail simulataneously: the action potential is prolonged, there is bradycardia and there is a reduction in outward, repolarizing current. As repolarization proceeds in these settings, any abnormal increase in net inward current may overcome the repolarization process causing a small depolarization. EADs usually occur near the end of the action potential plateau in a voltage range (window) likely to activate $I_{Ca,L}$. If this current is large enough to overcome the repolarization process, a significant depolarization will occur that can result in triggering of more SR Ca^{2+} release and an aftercontraction. This type of afterdepolarization can initiate a form of ventricular tachycardia called torsades de pointes.

- DADs are most frequently observed under conditions in which cytoplasmic $[Ca^{2+}]$ and SR Ca^{2+} content are increased. DADs take place during the diastolic interval distinct from any membrane potential changes associated with the action potential. They are caused by activation of Ca^{2+}-dependent currents following spontaneous releases of Ca^{2+} from the SR. The release of Ca^{2+} into the cytoplasm activates the Na^+/Ca^{2+} exchange and, in some species, Ca^{2+}-activated Cl^- current ($I_{Cl,Ca}$). The release of Ca^{2+} often causes an aftercontraction and the inward currents depolarize the cell. If the depolarizations are large enough they may reach a voltage range that will start to activate Na^+ channels and a premature action potential may result.

- The purpose of using anti-arrhythmic medication is to restore normal cardiac rhythm and rate and prevent the formation of dangerous arrhythmias. There are several ways these goals can be achieved: (1) altering the conduction velocity, (2) altering cell excitability by changing the duration of the ERP and (3) suppressing abnormal automaticity.

9.6 Questions

(1) Describe the terms "ectopic" and "automaticity" with reference to the heart.

(2) Describe the way excitation propagates along a single strand of cells.

(3) Contrast the formation of EADs with DADs.

(4) Describe the structure of gap junctions.

9.7 Bibliography

9.7.1 *Books and Reviews*

Kleber, A.G. and Rudy, Y. (2004). Basic mechanisms of cardiac impulse propagation and associated arrhythmias. *Physiol. Rev.* **84**, 431–488.

Kodama, I., Kamiya, K. and Toyama, J. (1997). Cellular electropharmacology of amiodarone. *Cardiovasc. Res.* **35**, 13–29.

Opie, L.H. (1995). *Drugs for the Heart* (4th edn). Saunders.

Volders, P.G., Vos, M.A., Szabo, B. *et al* (2000). Progress in the understanding of cardiac early afterdepolarizations and torsades de pointes: time to revise current concepts. *Cardiovasc. Res.* **46**, 376–392.

9.7.2 *Papers*

Fast, V.G. and Kleber, A.G. (1995). Cardiac tissue geometry as a determinant of unidirectional conduction block: assessment of microscopic excitation spread by optical mapping in patterned cell cultures and in a computer model. *Cardiovasc. Res.* **29**, 697–707.

Rohr, S., Kucera, J.P., Fast, V.G. and Kleber, A.G. (1997). Paradoxical improvement of impulse conduction in cardiac tissue by partial cellular uncoupling. *Science* **275**, 841–844.

Vaughan Williams, E.M. (1984). A classification of antiarrhythmic actions reassessed after a decade of new drugs. *J. Clin. Pharm.* **24**, 129–147.

Glossary of Electrophysiological Terms

Action potential: The transient electrical potential variation within a cell that is the physical basis of the nerve or muscle cell impulse.

Activation: Opening of a channel caused by a gating signal which can be produced by the presence of a ligand, a voltage change or a mechanical stimulus.

Active transport: Movement of ions or molecules against a concentration and/or electrical gradient by a mechanism that requires the expenditure of energy.

Anion: An atom or molecule in which the total number of electrons is greater than the total number of protons, giving it a net negative electrical charge.

Anisotropy: The directional variations of certain properties of propagation notably conduction velocity.

Bradycardia: A term describing a number of different conditions in which the heart beats at an unusually slow rate.

Capacitance: A measure of the ability of a substance to store charge. It can be defined by how much charge needs to be transferred between two conductors separated by an insulator to produce a potential difference between the conductors. Capacitance is denoted by C. The SI unit of capacitance is the farad (F). A capacitor of 1 farad with 1 volt across its conductors has +1 coulomb of charge stored on one conductor and −1 coulomb on the other.

Cation: An atom or molecule in which the total number of protons is greater than the total number of electrons, giving it a net positive electrical charge.

Charge: A property of matter that causes it to experience a force when close to other electrically charged matter. Charge is denoted by the symbol Q. The SI unit of charge is the coulomb (C). The electrical charge carried by a single proton is termed the elementary charge and is denoted by the symbol e. $e = 1.602 \times 10^{-19}$ coulombs.

Conductance: A measure of the ease with which current can flow between two points. Conductance is denoted by the symbol G and is measured in siemens (S). It is the reciprocal of resistance.

Conductivity: The degree to which a substance can pass current (or heat).

Current: The rate of flow of a charged species. Current is denoted by the symbol I and is measured in amperes or amps (A). One ampere is the flow of one coulomb of charge past a point in one second.

Current density: The electric current per unit of area. In the case of cells, the current measured from the whole cell is divided by the total capacitance of the cell, which is a measure of membrane area.

Deactivation: Closing of a channel due to the removal of a gating signal.

Depolarize: The term given to a reduction in the charge difference across the cell membrane. Often the term given to changes of membrane potential in the positive direction.

Desensitization: Closing of a ligand-gated channel when the activating ligand is still present.

Electrogenic: The term given to a process that transports charged particles in an asymmetrical way to create a potential difference across a membrane.

Excitation–contraction coupling: The mechanisms involved in muscle cells that link the electrical (excitatory) event with the mechanical (contraction) event.

Gating: Conformational changes in an ion channel induced by either ligand binding, trans-membrane voltage change or mechanical stimuli.

Gating current: A current resulting from the movement of charges associated with trans-membrane elements of ion channel proteins.

Hyperpolarize: The term given to an increase in the charge difference across the cell membrane. Often the term given to changes of membrane potential in the negative direction.

Inactivation: Closing of a channel in the continued presence of a gating signal.

Myocyte: A muscle cell.

Ohm's law: Named after the German physicist Georg Ohm and is a description of the relationship between voltage, current and resistance. $V = I \times R$.

Patch clamp: A form of voltage clamping by which a patch of membrane can be clamped. If the channel of interest is contained in the patch of membrane then one can record its behaviour in response to voltage or other stimuli.

Permeability: A measure of the ease with which a channel allows the passage of an ion.

Permeable: A channel state that allows an ion to move through it.

Permeant: The name given to a species capable of moving through a channel.

Rectification (applied to a channel): A term applied to a channel when the relationship between current flowing through it and the voltage applied across it is not linear, i.e. the conductance of the channel varies with voltage. Analogous to the electrical property that allows current to flow more easily in one direction than another.

Repolarize: The term associated with the return of membrane potential to a "resting" value.

Resistance: A measure of the opposition to the passage of current between two points. Resistance is denoted by the symbol R and is measured in ohms (Ω). The inverse of conductance.

Resistivity: The degree to which a substance resists the passage of current through it. The inverse of conductivity.

Selectivity: A measure of how well a channel allows an ion to pass through it while excluding other ions. Selectivity can be expressed as a permeability ratio.

Tachyarrhythmia: A disturbance of heart rhythm in which the heart rate is abnormally increased.

Tail current: A current that flows during the repolarizing phase of an action potential or voltage clamp command.

Voltage: The potential difference between two points or the work required to move a charge between the two points. Voltage is equivalent to potential difference. Voltage is denoted by V and potential difference is usually denoted by the symbol E. Membrane potential is denoted by E_m.

Answers to Chapter Questions

Chapter 2

(1) $E_m = 61 \log((1.5 \times 4) + (0.01 \times 140))/((1.5 \times 120) + (0.01 \times 10))$
$= -85$ mV

(2) $E_m = 61 \log ((1 \times 4) + (15 \times 140) + (0.1 \times 22))/((1 \times 120) + (15 \times 140) + (0.1 \times 100)) = 65$ mV

(3) -29 mV

Chapter 3

(1) Conductance depends on membrane potential, type and concentration of ion whereas permeability depends on membrane potential and the type of the ion in question.

(2) The inactivation process is a function of voltage and time. In Na^+ channels the inactivation process takes longer to occur than activation. When channels are inactivated they remain shut despite the membrane still being depolarized. Repolarization of the membrane is required to remove the inactivation and return the channels to a closed state from which they can be activated.

(3) (a)   True
    (b)   True
    (c)   True
    (d)   False – flow through Na^+ channels is also time dependent
    (e)   False – Na^+
    (f)   False – K^+
    (g)   True

Chapter 4

(1) Measure the macroscopic current (I_{ion}) and the microscopic (i_{ion}) current at the same voltage. Find the probability of the ion channels being open at that particular voltage. Then $P_{open} = (t_{open})/\text{total time}$). N = the number of active channels = $I_{ion}/(i_{ion} \times P_{open})$.

(2) Remember from Chapter 3 that V_{half} in the Na^+ channel activation curve is about −15 mV and assume that E_{Na} = +50 mV).

$i = \gamma \times (V_m - E_{Na}) = 30 \text{ pS} \times 65 \text{ mV} = 1950 \times 10^{-15} \text{ A} = 1.95 \text{ pA}$

Use the equation $I = i \times N$ where N is the number of active channels, i is the current through a single channel and I is the total current. $N_{tot} = N \times P_o$; at V_{half} $P_o = 0.5$.

Therefore: 2 nA = 1.95 pA $\times N$. Solving for N, we see that this cell has 1025 Na^+ channels. N_{tot} = 2050 channels.

(3) $P_o = 0.20$

(4) Driving force = 30mV
$\gamma = i/(V_m - E_{cation})$ (microscopic conductance = microscopic current/driving force)
100 pS = i/30 mV
i = 3.3 pA
$Q = I \times 0.2$ s (charge in coulombs (C) = current × seconds)
$Q = 3.3 \times 10^{-12}$ A $\times 0.2$ s = 6.6×10^{-13} C
1 coulomb contains 6.2×10^{18} elementary charges
$(6.6 \times 10^{-13}$ C$) \times (6.2 \times 10^{18}) = 4.09 \times 10^6$ ions in 200 ms

(5) Presence (or concentration) of the ligand and activation and inactivation kinetics of the channel.

Chapter 5

(1) Channels show gating and move ions rapidly (tens of millions per second per channel). Ion movement through a channel always results in net charge movement.

Active transporters do not show gating and transport ions less rapidly (hundreds per second per transporter). Ion movement may be electroneutral or electrogenic. While pumps or ATPases use ATP to help move ions against their concentration gradient, exchangers generally do not require ATP as an energy source.

(2) -47 mV

(3) These compounds inhibit the Na^+ pump which leads to an increase in intracellular $[Na^+]$. The increase in intracellular $[Na^+]$ pushes the exchange to more Ca influx and less Ca efflux during the cycle; intracellular $[Ca^{2+}]$ increases and so contraction becomes more powerful.

(4) -12 mV

(5) Since H^+ and Ca^{2+} share common buffering sites then these will bind H^+ and release Ca^{2+} in a reciprocal manner. The acidosis will activate the Na^+/H^+ exchange and Na^+/HCO_3^- symport leading to an increase in intracellular $[Na^+]$ which pushes NCX to more Ca^{2+} influx and less Ca^{2+} efflux during the cardiac cycle.

Chapter 6

(1) Unlike EC coupling in the heart, which requires influx of extracellular Ca^{2+} via the L-type channel, skeletal muscle EC coupling does not require Ca^{2+} influx. Transmission of the EC coupling signal from the voltage-sensing S4 regions of the skeletal DHPR to the pore of the skeletal form of RyR (RyR1)

depends on a conformational coupling between these two channels.

(2) They allow propagation of excitation into the cell to cause synchronous activation of RyRs ensuring spatially and temporally synchronous Ca^{2+} release throughout the cell. Secondly, many of the proteins involved in cellular Ca^{2+} cycling are concentrated at the T-tubule. Thirdly, changes in T-tubule structure and protein expression occur during the development of heart failure and this may be important in the decline of Ca^{2+} transient and contraction observed in these conditions.

(3) E_{Na} would be 70 mV. Na^+ channel inactivation and activation of early outward currents in the form of I_{to} can prevent the membrane potential from reaching E_{Na} and curtail the upstroke amplitude.

(4) The channels contributing to I_{to} show N-type inactivation involving the classic "ball and chain" mechanism.

(5) VDI involves direct obstruction of the pore by the I–II loop with the speed of inactivation in part dependent on its mobility. The mobility is reduced by interaction with the β2 subunit or the C-terminal tail with the CI region. The C-terminal tail acts as a "brake" to VDI. When Ca^{2+} binds to CaM the brake is removed which speeds inactivation.

Chapter 7

(1) At potentials more negative than E_K a large amount of inward current flows through channels carrying I_{K1} but less current flows at more positive potentials. At membrane potentials more positive than about –60 mV fewer channels are activated and at about –20 mV all channels are closed. Therefore no I_{K1} flows during the early plateau preventing rapid termination of the action potential and a loss of K^+ from the cells. The inward

rectifiying channels through which I_{K1} flows lack the voltage sensor or S4 segment and as a result they are insensitive to membrane voltage. Their opening and closing is dictated by the presence of polyvalent cations spermine and spermidine or Mg^{2+} in the channels which block the movement of K^+. The binding and unbinding of these molecules is a voltage-dependent process.

(2) The diffusion rate for K^+ in the T-tubules is about nine times slower than in free solution, so following increases in heart rate or a period of ischaemia, K^+ ions accumulate in the confined spaces, producing cell depolarization because E_K becomes more positive. The depolarization causes inactivation of a portion of Na^+ channels so fewer Na^+ channels are available for activation and therefore less current is generated to form the upstroke of the action potential. The result is that the upstroke is smaller and less rapid. I_{K1} channels are localized in the T-tubules so are modulated by the local changes in $[K^+]_o$. The increase in $[K^+]_o$ increases the conductance of I_{K1}. Under this condition more Na^+ influx will be required to overcome the stronger repolarizing effect of the increased outward K^+ flux and so this further limits the size of the depolarizing upstroke and reduces its speed.

(3) I_{Kur} is present in the atria but largely absent in the ventricle, so drugs specifically targeting that current may provide a selective therapy for atrial fibrillation. Inhibition of I_{Kur} would prolong the atrial action potential thereby increasing the effective refractory period and reducing the chances of re-excitation. Block of the current would lead to a more positive early plateau potential and, depending on the voltage range, this may activate more $I_{Ca,L}$. This would increase Ca^{2+} influx and lead to an increase in atrial contraction.

(4) Two structural features of $K_{V11.1}$ seem to be responsible for an array of drug interactions. The Pro-X-Pro sequence usually induces a kink in the S6 domain producing a small inner cavity

but the $K_{V11.1}$ channel lacks this sequence so there is no corresponding kink in S6. The $K_{V11.1}$ channel therefore has a larger inner cavity which can allow larger molecules access to binding sites. The two aromatic residues, tyrosine and phenylalanine, at 652 and 656 also appear important for drug binding.

(5) Slow Ca^{2+} release from the SR would result in a prolonged action of the Na^{+}/Ca^{2+} exchange in the forward (Ca^{2+} efflux) mode. This brings positive depolarizing charge into the cell which may prolong the action potential.

Chapter 8

(1) The unstable resting membrane potential in SA nodal cells is due to a lack of I_{K1}. The conductance of channels that produce I_{K1} is large so other currents also need to be large to change the membrane potential. Cells with I_{K1} tend to have stable resting membrane potentials. SA nodal cells express very few K_{ir} channels so that small changes in other currents flowing across the membrane can produce large changes in membrane potential.

(2) I_f is unusual because at physiologically relevant potentials it is an inward current that becomes larger as the cells are hyperpolarized. It activates on hyperpolarization from around -45 mV and deactivates rapidly upon depolarization to more positive voltages. These voltage ranges are modulated by the main neurotransmitters in the heart. These properties help in the generation of a slowly developing diastolic depolarization.

(3) The presence of β-receptor agonists increases the rate of diastolic depolarization and the presence of ACh slows the rate. Binding of noradrenaline to β-receptors increases the production of cAMP, which shifts the voltage dependence of HCN channel activation to more positive membrane potentials and thereby increases the number of open channels at any one voltage.

Therefore the rate of depolarization becomes faster which, in turn, increases heart rate. When ACh binds to muscarinic receptors the production of cAMP decreases. With less cAMP, the activation curve shifts to the left (more negative potentials) and so decreases the number of open channels at a given voltage. Under these conditions less depolarizing current flows and so the rate of depolarization is slower.

(4) This is the hypothesis that rhythmic intracellular Ca^{2+} oscillations generate the final part of the depolarization sequence that triggers the SA nodal action potential and has therefore been termed the "Ca^{2+} clock". Spontaneous and rhythmical local releases of SR Ca^{2+} ("Ca^{2+} wavelets") reach a peak late in the diastolic depolarization phase. They are accompanied by increases in inward current of the same periodicity. Lakatta and colleagues developed the view that these spontaneous Ca^{2+} release events are expelled from the nodal cells by the Na^+/Ca^{2+} exchange which, in so doing, generates an inward current. They propose that this inward current is responsible for accelerating the final phase of the diastolic depolarization leading to activation of the L-type Ca^{2+} channels and the action potential upstroke.

Chapter 9

(1) Any area of the heart that initiates impulses independently from the SA node is termed an ectopic focus. In order to produce pacemaker activity the focal area must have automaticity, i.e. be capable of producing independent excitation. Ectopic foci can result from hypoxic or ischaemic insults to the tissue, sympathetic overstimulation, enlargement of cells, slowing of the normal intrinsic heart rate, electrolyte disturbances and drug actions.

(2) Excitation of the cell at one end of the strand causes a small current to flow from this point source to the neighbouring cells

which are sinks of current. The current flow depends on the cytoplasmic and gap junctional resistances and results in a passive decay of voltage along the strand which is not propagated. If the active cell depolarizes its neighbouring cell sufficiently for it to reach its threshold potential then an action potential will be generated in that cell. If threshold is not reached then insufficient Na$^+$ channels will be activated, an action potential will not be evoked and propagation will cease.

(3) EADs tend to occur when several situations prevail simulataneously: the action potential is prolonged, there is bradycardia and there is a reduction in outward, repolarizing current. As repolarization proceeds in these settings, any abnormal increase in net inward current may overcome the repolarization process causing a small depolarization. EADs usually occur near the end of the action potential plateau in a voltage range (window) likely to activate $I_{Ca,L}$. If this current is large enough to overcome the repolarization process, a significant depolarization will occur which can result in triggering of more SR Ca^{2+} release and an aftercontraction. This type of afterdepolarization can initiate a form of ventricular tachycardia called torsades de pointes.

DADs are most frequently observed under conditions in which cytoplasmic [Ca^{2+}] and SR Ca^{2+} content are increased. DADs take place during the diastolic interval distinct from any membrane potential changes associated with the action potential. They are caused by activation of Ca^{2+}-dependent currents following spontaneous releases of Ca^{2+} from the SR. The release of Ca^{2+} into the cytoplasm activates the Na$^+$/Ca^{2+} exchange and, in some species, Ca^{2+}-activated Cl$^-$ current ($I_{Cl,Ca}$). The release of Ca^{2+} often causes an aftercontraction and the inward currents depolarize the cell. If the depolarizations are large enough they may reach a voltage range that will start to activate Na$^+$ channels and a premature action potential may result.

(4) Clusters of gap junctions form at intercalated discs and where the plasma membrane of the adjacent cell runs in close contact (gap of 2 nm). Each gap junction is formed from a cluster of connexons with each channel consisting of two connexons and each connexon of six connexins.

Index

3'-4'-dichlorobenzamil, 203
4-aminopyridine (4-AP), 149, 187, 221
9AC, 150

absolute refractory period, 137–139,
  174
acetylcholine, 77, 209, 211, 214–215,
  221
acidosis, 125
  effect on force, 124–125
action potential
  phases, 132–133
activation
  process, nerve, 48
activation variable
  m, 51
  n, 49
active transporters 106
adenosine, 245
A-kinase anchoring protein (AKAP),
  171
Aldrich, R., 97
alternative splicing, 75
amiloride, 122, 202
amiodarone, 189, 244, 249
ampere, 36
anatomy, 7
anisotropy, 231
apex, 8
Armstrong, C., 62, 87, 89, 97
arrhythmias, 225, 233–234, 240, 244,
  248
atrial fibrillation, 188–189, 243, 245,
  247
atrioventricular groove, 8
atrioventricular ring, 11
axon, 40

β-blockers, 245
ball and chain mechanism, 97, 146
base, 8
Bernstein, J., 3
BEST gene, 149
Bezanilla, F., 89
Brown, H., 211
bundle branch block, 237
Burdon Sanderson, J., 4

Ca^{2+} channel
  alpha interaction domain, 162
  beta interaction domain, 162
  conduction, 164
  EEEE domain, 165
  IQ calmodulin-binding motif, 168
  L-type, 131–132, 156–160, 163, 166,
    169, 170–171
  mole fraction, 165
  regulation, 169, 170–171
  structure, 162, 175
  T-type, 160
Ca^{2+} current, 152
  blocking agents, 242
  facilitation, 169, 175
  inactivation, 166–168, 175
  L-type, 149, 151–153, 166, 171–172,
    174, 218, 227,
    activation, 152
    reversal potential, 153
    role in EC coupling, 153
  LVA, 216
  N-type, 160
  sub-types, 161
  T-type, 172, 216, 218–219
Ca^{2+} sparks, 157–158, 175
Ca^{2+} transient, 156–157, 164, 175
Ca^{2+} wavelets, 218